Mental Disease in History

The Reshaping of Psychoanalysis From Sigmund Freud to Ernest Becker

Barry R. Arnold
General Editor

Vol. 7

PETER LANG
New York • Washington, D.C./Baltimore
Bern • Frankfurt am Main • Berlin • Vienna • Paris

Mental Disease in History

A Selection of Translated Readings

Edited by
J. Thomas Dalby

PETER LANG
New York • Washington, D.C./Baltimore
Bern • Frankfurt am Main • Berlin • Vienna • Paris

Library of Congress Cataloging-in-Publication Data

Mental disease in history: a selection of
translated readings/ J. Thomas Dalby, editor.
p. cm. — (Reshaping of psychoanalysis; v. 7)
1. Mental illness—History. 2. Schizophrenia—History.
I. Dalby, J. Thomas (John Thomas). II. Series.
RC454.4.M455 616.89'009—dc20 96-33891
ISBN 0-8204-3056-0
ISSN 1059-3551

Die Deutsche Bibliothek-CIP-Einheitsaufnahme

Mental disease in history: a selection of translated readings/ J. Thomas Dalby, editor. –New York; Washington, D.C./Baltimore; Bern; Frankfurt am Main; Berlin; Vienna; Paris: Lang.
(The reshaping of psychoanalysis; Vol. 7)
ISBN 0-8204-3056-0
NE: Dalby, J. Thomas [Hrsg.];GT

Cover design by James F. Brisson.

Dedication

This book is dedicated to the memory of Lloyd Wilfred Bebensee (1927 - 1996). In 1984 Lloyd and his wife Elaine established a registered charitable foundation to support research into the causes and treatments of schizophrenia. He was a man of clear integrity, creative intelligence and unrelenting determination. I will miss my frequent discussions with him on myriad topics, his personal warmth and his overriding optimism that those afflicted with mental diseases would, one day, be freed from their manacles.

Acknowledgments

I would like to extend my thanks to the Ian Douglas Bebensee Foundation for their generous support of this project. In particular, I would like to extend my appreciation for the constant encouragement provided by foundation members Lloyd Bebensee and Jack Stewart.

The primary translation of articles was conducted by Krista Dalby (French), Isidro Moreira (Spanish) and Natasha Johnson (German) with final translation decisions by the editor. Word processing of the manuscript was performed by Meagan Dalby.

I would like to thank the copyright holders (publishers and/or authors) for permission to translate and reprint these articles. The original references are cited as follows:

J. P. Gueguen, Histoire du concept de schizophrénie. Soins Psychiatrie, 1988, 89, 4-6. (©INTEREDITIONS, Paris)

W. Janzarik, Geschichte und problematik des schizophreniebegriffes. Der Nervenarzt, 1986, 57, 681-685.

C. Scharfetter, Streifzüge in die Geschichte des Schizophreniebegriffs. Schweizer Archiv für Neurologie, Neurochirurgie und Psychiatrie, 1973, 112, 75-85.

L. E. Bellomo, El defecto esquizofrenico. Acta Psiquiátrica y Psicol—gica de América Latina, 1987, 33, 305-315.

E. A. Gomez, El problema del enfermo mental cr—nico indigente: un análisis hist—rico. Acta Psiquiátrica y Psicol—gica de América Latina, 1983, 29, 213-222.

D. Moreau, Peur et folie. Soins Psychiatrie, 1988, 92/93, 9-14. (©INTEREDITIONS, Paris)

J. Alliez, J.-P. Huber, L'acédie ou le déprimé entre le péché et la maladie. Annales Médico-Psychologiques, 1987, 145, 393-407.

M. Henne, La schizophrénie n'est plus ce qu'elle était. Annales Médico-Psychologiques, 1979, 137, 256-260.

M. Bleuler, Zur entstehung und bedeutung von Eugen Bleulers werk: "Dementia praecox oder gruppe der schizophrenien". Schweizerische Rundschau Fuer Medizin (PRAXIS) 77, 48, 1322-1326.

C. Scharfetter, Psychische vulnerabilität - Canstatt 1841. Der Nervenarzt, 1987, 58, 527.

U. H. Peters, Die deutsche schizophrenielehre und die psychiatrische emigration. Fortschritte der Neurologie, Psychiatrie, 1988, 56, 347-360.

E. La Croce, El concepto de locura en Grecia clásica. Acta Psiquiátrica y Psicol—gica de América Latina, 1981, 27, 285-291.

C. Kläui, Vom irren armen zum armen irren: Eine untersuchung zu irrenwesen und irrsinn im barocken Rom. Gesnerus, 1986, 43, 279-298.

M. Granek, Le concept de fou et ses implications dans la litterature Talmudique et ses exegeses. Annales Médico-Psychologiques, 1976, 134, 17-35.

F. P. Larraya, Locura y hechiceria en la inquisicion del Rio de la Plata, Acta Psiquiátrica y Psicol—gica de América Latina, 1988, 34, 211-222.

F. Furukawa, M. Bourgeois, Délires de possession par le renard au Japon (ou délire de Kitsune-Tsuki). Annales Médico-Psychologiques, 1984, 142, 677-687.

C. Müller, Historische reminiszenz: die schizophrene psychose der Kaiserin von Mexiko. Fortschritte der Neurologie, Psychiatrie, 1979, 47, 550-552.

J. E. Meyer, R. Meyer, Selbstzeugnisse eines schizophrenen um 1800. Confinia Psychiatrica, 1969, 12, 130-143.

Contents

Preface

In my research on the history of mental disorders I would continually come across vague and intriguing references to articles in foreign languages which were not easily accessible. With the aid of the Ian Douglas Bebensee Foundation - an organization devoted to the support of research into schizophrenia - I was able to obtain and translate, with substantial assistance from others whose command of these tongues was far superior to my rather primitive skill, a series of papers which explored various aspects of the history of mental disease. Translating words and ideas is an arduous task, for there are occasions when a direct parallel is awkward or unavailable. We have tried to stay as close to the original authors' thoughts rather than rewrite or reinterpret (to any large degree) their work. It seemed selfish to relegate these gems to my private archives so I selected a sample for dissemination which offered information not readily available in English or presented a fresh perspective on issues.

In front of you is a smorgasbord of international offerings. Like all buffets you may find a few things not particular to your interests or tastes but it is probable that if you look carefully you can find some satisfaction of your appetite for this type of history. Some of the pieces are light appetizers, others more conducive to a main course and some are pleasant deserts. I hope that they nourish your intellect and whet the creative palate, for the knowledge of our past can guide us in our modern investigations and theories.

Enjoy!

J. Thomas Dalby, Ph.D.
Calgary, Alberta, Canada
February 1996

Introduction

Volume Seven by Dr. Thomas Dalby is an exceptionally fine contribution to my series *The Reshaping of Psychoanalysis: From Sigmund Freud to Ernest Becker.* Volume one offered a purist interpretation of Freudian theory against the revisionists. Volume two presented an existential/ phenomenological approach to disease with some appreciation of potential rapprochement between psychoanalysis and itself. Volume three presented a portrayal of Ernest Becker's seminal contributions to psychoanalytic theory while offering interstitial connections with transactional analysis. Volume four concentrated on the psychoanalytic contributions of Campbell and Jung, underscoring the potential meshing of depth psychology, psychoanalysis, and spirituality. Volume five creatively elucidated the positivity and negativity associated with the multifaceted contributions of psychopharmacology. Volume six pioneered new psychological territory by seeking a bridge between varied 'anti-establishment' psychologies, giving particularly illuminative studies of radical groups such as EST. Volume seven now brings to light some very important works on such topics as schizophrenia, madness, acedia, among others which because of language barriers had been virtually lost to the English speaking psychological/ psychiatric community. These works are especially valuable because they exposit historical antecedents to modern psychiatric theory. In a very real sense, they offer the delineation of a much needed historical context to help us sense the long, often convoluted, even tortuous pathway to psychiatry at the close of the twentieth century. Further, the selections are not only astutely translated but quite well chosen in their ability to remind those of us in the psychological/ psychiatric community of an exceptionally variegated past history.

If I may, I would like to underscore my own understanding of the psychological problem of modernity which gave rise to this series as a whole.

Characterizing modern humanity via diagnostic labels such as "anxiety" is pervasive throughout the literature of most any field. It is significant to elucidate the anxious state of the human in order to underscore and intensify our understanding of the plight of the modern human. The human's own ambiguity in an ambiguous situation is vivified in narcissism, e.g., for the self continually senses its own impotence, its own emptiness. In its narcissism, the self realizes he must focus on himself while simultaneously recognizing that he really cannot rely upon himself. He is insufficient. With Rollo May, such a recognition of insufficiency brings anxiety as a "threat to some value which the individual holds essential to his existence as a personality."[1] With Karen Horney, anxiety becomes "a generalized sense of helplessness, a sense that the fundamental powers to resolve contradictory tendencies are lost."[2] Anxiety becomes obsessive because the self knows that the construct, the frame of reference out of which his being operated, is facing dissolution; and he knows that he must create some mechanism for survival. His deracinated self attempts to form the construct in "mid-air, in vacuo." Nothing from nothing yields nothing. The self as ego is dysfunctional, for its narcissism allows no external object to which it may relate and from which it may learn. "...ego functioning consists precisely in... organizing the discharge of instincts upon objects."[3] The narcissistic individual faces anxiety because the dysfunctional ego has only its ambiguous, undirected energies with which to deal. The self simply percolates, teeming with its own energies. The potentialities for self-destruction are limitless. "...in the presence of dammed-up libido, the acute signal often has the same effect as a match in a barrel of gunpowder... the ego, in giving a signal, has set off something which... it can no longer control.[4] The self, fragmented in its ontological deracination surging for answers, for stability in an anxiety-ridden *Sitz im Leben*, is certainly volatile. The directionless self seethes anxiously until such energies may be directed/ canalized appropriately. During the interim, the ego must provide some semblance of order in an executive fashion to the drive energies pressing for discharge.[5] A cramped, fearful, profoundly anxious self is what is left for such execution.

The anxious, narcissistic self of modernity searches for direction but with no map, no blueprint other than one of his own creation; and it necessarily yields no light for the way because his map can reflect no more than his own "lostness." He remains alone in his alienation and anxiety.

> Each person, withdrawn into himself, behaves as though he is a stranger to the destiny of all the others. His children and his good friends constitute for him the whole the human species. As for his transactions with his fellow citizens, he may mix among them but he sees them not; he touches them but does not feel them; he exists only in himself and for himself alone.[6]

Staying "afloat" within this narcissistic *Weltanschauung* is as problem, for propensities toward psychopathology are operating at every turn. The totally free self, drowning in its lack of definition, its ambiguity, may find its loneliness, its alienation, its anxiety too problematic. Without the thread of Ariadne, the guide rope, to follow into and out of one's madness,[7] the self may find itself "teetering on the psychotic edge..."[8]

Woody Allen's 1983 motion picture, *Zelig* vividly portrays what we have designated as the anxious, floating, boundariless, borderline, deracinated personality. Allen, admittedly, in his typical satirical style is giving a comedic twist to this illumination of the fictitious character of Leonard Zelig, a 1929 psychotic. Still, the characterology of a human being lost in a variety of roles remains bitingly sober since Zelig's lostness encapsulates everyman's lostness in a society coercing the *status quo* and conformity. Astoundingly yet appropriately, Allen utilizes the comment of psychoanalyst Bruno Bettelheim in his script as Bettelheim characterizes Zelig via an interview "as the ultimate conformist."[9] Another character at-large comments "he wanted to assimilate like crazy."[10] The medical community identifies him as a "human chameleon"[11] who "protects himself by becoming whoever he's around."[12] Allen's buffoonery has Zelig become a national star because of his medical uniqueness resulting in a dance being named after him-- "doing the chameleon."[13]

Able descriptions of the characterology still permeate the chicanery. Allen has Folies Bergere star Josephine Baker see Zelig as "amazing but a little lost."[14] In a more comedic vein, Allen has Zelig clothe his meaningless and his lack of a stable tradition in stand-up comedy material. "I run into a synagogue - I ask the Rabbi the meaning of life -- he tells me the meaning of life but he tells it to me in Hebrew -- I don't understand Hebrew -- then he wants to charge me $600 for Hebrew lessons."[15] Similarly, Zelig's father indicated to Leonard from his deathbed that "life is a meaningless nightmare of suffering."[16] The commentator continues "...the only advice that he gives him is to save string."[17] Appropriately, we find out that in the same context that Leonard's brother Jack is a victim of "a nervous breakdown"[18] and that "sister Ruth becomes a shoplifter."[19]

From a psychiatrist one finds a good description of Zelig's plight explicated more technically: "somewhere behind that vacuous face, that zombie like stare is a real human being."[20] Another commentator states perhaps the finest explication of the deracinated human as he says of Zelig:

> Zelig's own existence is nonexistence, devoid of personality--quietly staring into space, a cipher, a performing freak-- he who wanted only to fit in, to belong, to go unseen by his enemies and be loved-- neither fits in or belongs.[21]

Even Zelig himself has some inkling of his tragic plight as he answers certain questions from his psychiatrist. She asks, "Tell me why you assume the characteristics of the person you're with?"[22] He replies, "it's safe"... "I want to be liked."[23] Finally confronted with himself, Zelig at one point whimpers in melancholia, "I'm nobody. I'm nothing. Catch me, I'm falling."[24]

Zelig is most poignant in his character when he conquers his malady and realizes what a true human being must be. "...you have to be your own person and make your own moral choices even when they do require courage; otherwise you're like a robot or a lizard."[25] With the help of his loyal psychiatrist, Zelig is able to analyze, i.e., see through himself and his malady, and move toward full recovery. In the analysis he senses those attributes of character necessary to being human such as courage, self-expression, and moral decision-making. The malady forces an insightful evaluation which would have been completely unknown without the forced tragedy of the pathology. Perhaps this is what Saul Bellow is saying when Allen has him state of Zelig in an interview "...therefore his sickness was also at the root of his salvation."[26]

Certainly there is much more to this film than I have elucidated. Allen's humor moves through Hitler to upside down airplane rides across the Atlantic. Zelig regresses and gets well again. None of these events preclude the general point I am making and which I believe Allen is making. The chameleon personality which takes on roles with no real investment in them other than security reasons is the paradigmatic characterology of our present time period. This chameleon personality is a non-entity, an onion without a core, a being without roots, without discretion, without self. As Stanley Kauffmann puts it, "...we can take him as a metaphor for our century's pressures on individuality, diabolically counterpointed by the growth of hype."[27]

The percolating anxieties may lead to his floating, percolating kind of madness in which the self simply loses its identity definition; or it may lead to a defensive imprisoning of the self. The ego imprisonment occurs, because the self accepts any structure in order to avoid the ambiguities of the "floating" madness and fails to realize that the new, ordered self is but a caged madness.

Max Weber prognosticates this twentieth century predicament. In *The Protestant Ethic and the Spirit of Capitalism*, Weber sees the "mighty cosmos of the modern economic order as 'an iron cage'."[28] And "not only is modern society a cage, but all the people in it are shaped by its bars; we are beings without spirit, without heart, without sexual or personal identity..."[29] The overly structured selves via a superimposed economic structure are not identities but drones assembled for the assembly lines. Persons fit themselves to proper roles rather than creating identities for themselves within the economic frame of reference. Persons accept the constructs given to them in order to give some definition or parameters to the deracinated self. The efficacy, the workability of such a construct must inevitably stand the test of the Marxian psychology, "all that is solid melts into air." Weberians seem to indicate that cages are the most apt to melt. Psychopathology is clothed in socioeconomic or sociopolitical jargon; it remains, nonetheless, disease. Attempting to create stability and solidity in a partialized fashion by holding to the economic delimitation of identity results in a narrow, neurotic self. The work of Otto Rank certainly helps one to see the devastating effects of such a narrowing, such a confining of the self.[30] With Jung, I envisage this new self as one foolishly seeking to "preserve a degree of integrity at the expense of over-all integrity."[31] A degree of integrity is a collective misnomer, for integrity must always mean the psychic integration in the whole person, bringing a "reasonable long-term integrity of the person as autonomous agent."[32] "Degree of integrity" simply indicates neurotic partialization. The self is sick in its confinement.

Endnotes

1. Herbert Fingarette, The Self in Transformation. Psychoanalysis, Philosophy and the Life of the Spirit (New York: Harper and Row, 1963),p. 88.

2. Ibid., p. 89.

3. Ibid., p. 76.

4. Ibid., p. 83.

5. Ibid., p. 75.

6. Richard Sennett, The Fall of Public Man (New York: Alfred A. Knopf, 1977), p. viii.

7. Sam Keen, Beginnings Without End (New York: Harper and Row Publishers, 1975), p. 70.

8. bid., p. 69.

9. Woody Allen, dir., Zelig (1983).

10. 26. Ibid.

27. Stanley Kauffmann, "One Character in Search of an Author," New Republic, 189 (August 15-22, 1983), p. 25.

28. Marshall Berman, All That is Solid Melts Into Air (Simon and Schuster, 1982), p. 27.

29. Ibid., p. 69.

30. See the Rankian Tendenz in Ernest Becker, The Denial of Death (New York: The Free Press, 1973), passim.

31. Herbert Fingarette, p. 90.

32. Ibid., p. 76.

Barry Arnold, Ph.D.
Milton, Florida
March 1996
Series Editor - *"The Reshaping of Psychoanalysis: From Sigmund Freud to Ernest Becker"*

History of the Concept of Schizophrenia

J. P. Gueguen

Summary: The term schizophrenia is a new one because it only appears for the first time in literature in 1911 under the pen of a Swiss psychiatrist in the German language: Eugen Bleuler (1857-1939).

History

UP UNTIL THE END of the 19th century, the psychiatric nosology was still quite sparse. Even so, Pinel (1745-1826), since 1800, spoke of acquired idiocy and his pupil, Esquirol (1772-1840), of insanity occurring before 25 years of age(1). These are all great theories that contradict one another, looking to find a universal explanation for mental illness.

This follows pseudo-scientific theories, such as the physiognomy of Lavater, the phrenology of Gall (the theory of bumps...) and, later on, Morel's (1809-1873) theory of degeneration, which was the first to speak of precocious insanity. In his 'clinical studies', he describes lunatics, still young, thus we can imagine they can be cured...

But this observation remains relatively isolated; Morel looks to relate everything to the concept of degeneration that he created and preoccupies, in this era, a preponderant place in the French school of psychiatry.

In effect, the only illness resting on clinical and anatomical-pathological bases remained, throughout the 19th century, general paralysis. This illness, described by Bayle (1799-1858), in 1825, for almost half a century, served as a model of reference and will mark the history of psychiatry for a long time (2).

The Concept of Schizophrenia

It is in the countries of the German language that the concept of schizophrenia would slowly take form.

Between 1863 and 1884, Kahlbaum and his pupil Hecker would, for the first attempt at classification of mental illness, describe hebephrenia (madness of youth) which hits young people at puberty and leads to insanity. Of this group, they isolate catatonia, the madness which is characterized by specific symptoms: inertia, loss of motor activity and catalepsy... Later, Kahlbaum describes an extenuated and curable form of hebephrenia which evolved under a psychopathic form: heboidophrenia.

But it wasn't until the end of the 19th century that German psychiatrist Emil Kraepelin would, through a rigorous clinical approach, found all the great nosographic frames, which even today provide a reference for us.

It is thus that he defines the concept of "Dementia praecox" that groups three clinical types: 'catatonia', 'hebephrenia', and the 'delirious' (paranoid) form (3).

The description of each of these forms is thus previous to Kraepelin; but we must give to the latter the merit of having regrouped them under a single clinical entity, thus the criteria are not only semeiological, but also evolutionary. Kraepelin's contemporaries note, in addition, that it acts not so much as insanity, in a weakened, intellectual sense, but a genuine disintegration of the personality (4).

Psychodynamic Conceptions

Eugen Bleuler (1857-1939) finally proposed an approach more psychodynamic than descriptive of mental illnesses, that would substitute the concept of dementia praecox for the concept of schizophrenia. "I call dementia praecox schizophrenia because the dislocation of the diverse psychic functions is one of its most important characteristics".

Bleuler, influenced in this by the psychodynamic conceptions of Freud and Jung, describes the primary symptoms (deficits) that constitute the pathological process, and the secondary symptoms, which begin only with reaction of diseased mind.

It opposes the fundamental syndrome, which constitutes the dissociation, the secondary symptoms which constitute a sort of 'reaction of the ill soul'. (Bleuler quoted by Postel) (3). Then, it's under the term autism that he describes the delirious break with reality. Now, this presents a new approach to mental pathology since the frenzy is no longer considered as a constituent of the illness, but as a reaction to the morbid underlying process.

In 1921, Kretschmer describes, in 'The structure of body and of character', a positive correlation between schizophrenia and the morphologic ectomorph type (tall and slender figure). This biotype, for him, corresponds to a schizothymic character, thus the pathological form would be schizoid (personality introverted, solitary and distant...) (5).

In France, Bleuler's theory was introduced by Trenel and above all, Minkowski, who insisted on the loss of vital contact with reality, leaving a bit to the side discord and dissociation. Henri Claude, in 1926, described the group of psychoses, whose form, at least, would be the schizoid constitution (1).

Afterwards, the concept of schizophrenia would be known as a great extension, in particular in Anglo-Saxon countries. Bleuler then speaks of 'group of schizophrenias', of which he excludes only manic-depressive psychosis, neuroses and organic processes.

The French psychiatrist, heir of a long tradition, prefers keeping a nosology more rigorous, excluding schizophrenia and chronic madness. And still today, our nosography occupies an important place in international literature.

That is what it was, we can say at the dawn of the Second World War, the clinical picture of schizophrenia is finally well-drawn, and the studies over the last fifty years would overall orient towards etiopathogeny and the therapeutic possibilities of the illness.

Therapeutic Possibilities -
Insulin therapy

Thus insulin therapy, discovered in the thirties by Sakel, would constitute the first tentative biological treatment of schizophrenia. Up to the appearance of neuroleptics in 1952, hypoglycemic shocks would be the principal treatment used for this disorder.

Electroconvulsive Therapy

Around the same time, the Hungarian Meduna would put to the point convulsive therapy by injection of metrazol. This method, of a difficult and dangerous operation, would rapidly give way in 1938 to shock therapy discovered by Cerletti, whose indicative type, since 1940, would be melancholy more than schizophrenia.

Sleeping Cures

Finally, signaling that sleeping cures had been praised by some, at the beginning of the sixties, the method of humid wrapping emerged. But these therapeutics would remain relatively marginal (2).

Neuroleptics

In effect, since 1952, with the discovery of chlorpromazine (Largactil), the neuroleptics occupied a major place in the treatment of this disease.

Starting in 1950, psychotherapies, be they analytical, institutional, individual or familial, become equally an essential element in taking charge of schizophrenics. The road was opened in 1929 by Simmel and Federn who were the first to propose a psychoanalytic approach to psychoses (4).

Etiopathogenesis

But no clinical picture could be complete if they didn't explain the causes and the process that determines the evolution of an illness.

Heredity

Since 1928, research concerning heredity has employed the schema of true twins. So the rate of concordance (which varies among authors) is found again each time, and no one could put into evidence a coherent schema of hereditary transmission. Now we speak of nothing other than 'hereditary predisposition', where the rate of risk is higher in certain families.

Neurobiological Studies

In the same fashion, anatomopathological and neurobiological studies do not have a definitive conclusion. In 1962, a dopaminergic theory of schizophrenia (the biochemical mechanism of the illness which is hypodopaminergic) gave great hopes, but rapidly became qualified...

Psychosocial Factors

The studies concerning psychosocial and familial factors equally occupied a preponderant place in this tentative explanation of the illness. For history, we cite the school of Palo Alto and the theory of double bind of Bateson, and turn next to England and Laing who described this double bind as 'an untenable position imposed on the schizophrenic subject" (Laing quoted by Ey) (4). This thesis, pushed to the extreme by Cooper, leads to the exclusively sociological theory of schizophrenia and blooms, in the sixties, into the anti-psychiatric movement.

Psychoanalysis

Certainly, psychoanalysis was never absent of debate, even though it tries to elaborate a theory more global than psychosis. It was Freud, at first, relayed by Bleuler and Jung, who proposed an analytical interpretation of these disorders. In fact, psychoanalysis has, above all, earned the merit of proposing more and more coherant psychopathological models which, inspiring all above the clinical, permits a better comprehension of schizophrenia and emerges into therapeutic propositions.

However, we can observe here the (relative) failure of all the tentative etiopathogenic explanations which reduced schizophrenia to a system of which etiology would be exclusively genetic, neurobiologic or psycho-sociological.

If the correlations could be recovered on the genetic plan, we could never prove the hereditary factor. If these anatamopathological and biological anomalies were equally proven with a certain number of schizophrenics, we could never determine if they would constitute the cause of the illness or if they only marked the evolutionary process. Psychoanalysis proposed the models of comprehension which rendered the discourse of schizophrenia less impenetrable, but only partially explains the reasons and origins.

In effect, if these theories posed the problem for an exogenous or endogenous process - and only reached to partially resolve it - they must not omit the interaction which forcibly exists between a subject, if he's ill, and his environment. This dialectic obliges us to take caution. It urges us to approach the individual in a global fashion in which no element could be detached. It designates mental illness as a resulting set, whose casualties, it is evident, cannot enter into a fixed monolithic system.

The dominant view of schizophrenics, anyhow, corroborates this hypothesis since their treatment is henceforth, more and more, multi-form.

Conclusion

We cannot end the history of schizophrenia without speaking of DSM III (Diagnostic and Statistical Manual of Mental Disorders), of American origin, the first edition dated 1952. Its aims are exclusively semeiologic and diagnostic. It intentionally ignores all psychopathological and etiologic sources and no longer searches to define the illness but to regroup the symptoms. It speaks not of schizophrenia, but of "schizophrenic disorders."

This approach, resolutely distanced and practically apprised of mental illness, may leave us indifferent. It has the merit to return the words back to their proper meaning. It redefines schizophrenia exclusively in relation to its symptoms. It reduces this pathology to no other, in erasing the evolutionary movement. But in stratifying, thus, that which dwells in an incredible complexity, it risks making us approach the patients with a fixation which has little to do with their personal history.

It remains thus, that this illness we can see, although the outlines are difficult to pinpoint, never stops us from questioning, with the same concept of mental illness, thus we know more if the successive descriptions correspond to well-defined entities or constitute the 'models' in perpetual evolution.❧

References

1. Guiraud P. - Origine et évolution de la notion de schizophrénie. Confrontations psychiatriques, 1968, 2: 9-29.

2. Pichot P. - Un siècle de psychiatrie. Paris, Ed. Roger Dacosta, 1983.

3. Postel J., Quetel C. - Historie de la psychiatrie. Toulosse, Privat, 1983.

4. Ey H., Bernard P., Brisset C. - Manuel de psychiatrie, 5e Ed., Paris, 1978: 534-69.

5. Lemperière T., Féline A. - Psychiatrie de l'adulte. Paris, Masson, 1981: 245-53.

6. American psychiatric association. - DSM III, Paris, Masson, 1983.

The Concept of Schizophrenia: Its History and its Problems

W. Janzarik

THE HISTORY OF SCHIZOPHRENIA is the history of the psychopathological syndrome, which was late to be understood under a new terminology after continuous new definitions and classifications. Fundamental problems of psychiatric theory resulted from dwelling on endogenous; functional or idiopathic psychoses and especially schizophrenia. Only certain sections of these two themes can be dealt with. Proceeding from the concept's history, certain questions arise concerning the psychiatric taxonomy, which are tied in with historical developments in the concept of schizophrenia.

New names and terms for illnesses appeared within the German language which would lead to dementia praecox and schizophrenia; for example is Snell's 1865 report (27) on "Monomania as a primary form of mental disturbance". Griesinger (8), who also referred to Morel in this regard, agreed with Snell. In 1867, in his report for the inauguration of the Berlin Clinic of "Primary Insanity", Griesinger used a synonymous term. Later, supported by his teacher, Zeller, he acknowledges only affective and reversible disorders as being primary. An illness process, he thought, to be unified can terminate in affective and schizoaffective disorders at a later time, with this affective type of illness. The illness process, however, can no longer progress to regressive weakness conditions with a damaging of thought and will.

Griesinger termed secondary developing conditions of weakness as "madness" and "imbecility" and described them as being encompassed in the sense of chronic schizophrenia. In 1867 Griesinger gave up the system of mental illness which had been standard for his time, with the assumption that insanity could develop without earlier provisions of melancholy and mania.

In the years after Griesinger's death (1868) a new encompassing clinical synthesis established itself on the grounds of "primary madness". In reading Sander (24) it is apparent that the majority of institutional patients were comprised of the insane and they formed the main topic of public mental care. Schüle (26) in 1878 saw nothing other than the earliest occurrences of madness in Kahlbaum's and Hecker's hebephrenia, Westphal (28) also classed Kahlbaum's "catatonic" illness here. Already in 1878 madness, as defined by Westphal, could be employed carrying equal meaning to the term schizophrenia.

The two decades separating the terms "madness" and "dementia praecox" were due to several reasons. A comprehensive image of this illness already existed whose description corresponded exactly to the later "dementia praecox". Therefore only a common lingual denotation existed, without a connecting scientific term, meaning that an author implying madness might also use the word insanity. In Griesinger's original wording and consequential clear conceptions, a loss of inner connection and regulated strength is seen after the widening of the limits of "primary madness". Its fragments would be further transformed into denotation of independent illnesses. The original conception of power also remained reduced to Kahlbaum's "vensania typica".

The consequences which could be drawn from a unified domain of affective disorders (coming from the 1850's with Falret's folie circulaire form and Baillarger's folie à deux) were not seen at this time. Since Griesinger's death madness and folie à deux form were seen as two opposing blocks preventing the development of diagnoses - without this view the Kraepelinian dichotomy in its brilliant simplicity would have been directly attainable much earlier. Since antiquity, antecedents to concepts of melancholy and mania had yet another meaning opposed to pure affective disturbances. "Melancholy" implied a partial mental disturbance and "mania" a generalized one, which was also possibly classed with "insanity". Through the classification of periodic developments during which the conceptions of melancholic and manic conditions became detached form each other, in the last third of the century, melancholy and mania were eventually narrowed to affective disorders. From there madness confronts an extensive and open catalogue of other mental illnesses. Because of his nosographical intentions, Kahlbaum directly blocked the way to an easy solution. Kraepelin followed him for a long time indirectly (15) with his concept of paranoia.

Thankfully, further observations of development offered favorable assumptions to the Heidelberg clinic; because of its institutional character of the time, Kraepelin could eventually establish a difference between feeling-illness and mental illness, providing relief to a terminology which had become chaotic. In the 6th edition of his 1899 (17) theory book, an inclusive meaning was obtained, following 1893's conception of "dementia praecox". Bleuler's term "schizophrenia" of 1908 (meaning the same as dementia praecox) (4) took over as a factually and linguistically improved term. After that, the semantic meaning between the two terms shifted.

The vicissitudes of the lines drawn between the two idiopathic areas of form should be outlined as part of the history of the concepts of schizophrenia because it leads to a central question. On the one hand, schizophrenics display characteristics of dementia praecox or a narrower definition has been created such as Kleist and Leonhards "systematic schizophrenia" and other examples where atypical reactive forms of schizophrenia and other special forms are differentiated from the core group. A very broad and latent schizophrenia exists on the other hand, which includes Bleuler's concept of the disease and the psychoanalysts of America ruling psychiatry for several decades. The middle line of psychopathology originating from K. Jaspers Heidelberg school and K. Schneider was closer to Bleuler and not Kraepelin's development theory and supported on psychopathologic phenomena of the primary rank symptoms. The inclusion of one defined the borders of the other. The much quoted work of Pope and Lipinski (23) (1978) gives an example of the last decade's neo-Kraepelinism again being turned back on a narrow frame of dementia praecox. Already, Kraepelin's student Wilmanns (29) along with J. Lange (20) had put affect-psychotic underlying psychoses with insanity, tricks of the senses and catatonic phenomena but without changing it to connect it with manic-depression. The DSM-III (6) classed manic and depressive episodes with mood-incongruent psychotic characteristics as well as with first rank symptoms as a typical affective disorder. In the succession after Wernicke, beginning with Kleist, Schröder and Leonhard, an attempt at narrowing diagnoses of schizophrenia was made, using other terminology such as schizoaffective diseases, paranoid disorders, psychotic disorders and paranoid/schizoaffective personality disorders.

A book could be written on the changing of the concept of schizophrenia over the century. However, no convincing advances were made toward a secured objective nosology. In the circle of idiopathic psychosyndromes, diagnoses are evidently conventions supported by psychopathological phenomena and development criteria which can neither be right nor wrong but reliable and functional. Diagnoses such as progressive paralysis or Huntington's Chorea which indicates a unity of illness in the original sense of nosological beginnings are exceptions. It appears that the majority of psychiatric diagnoses are based on theoretical preliminary decisions and methodological beginnings belonging to recognized conventions of the time. Not least, the momentary balance of power in the psychiatric industry is reflected in diagnoses.

The psychiatric system of the 20th century is Kraepelin's system even if the principle of its membership developed from a phantom. Kraepelin searched for and found unities of illness. It was derived from observation of development in Kahlbaum's sense and French Psychiatry as Pichot (22) remembered. It was certain that this would have the confirmation of neuropathology and a hope which remains. The illness model which was first supported by progressive paralysis and neurology with it's visual patterns of thought belongs to a one-sided biological consideration but also to the antithesis of an exclusive psychogenesis. K. Schneider (25) stressed the conventional character of psychiatric diagnostics; the psychopathological conventions termed "cyclothymia" and "schizophrenia" by him asserted a somatic illness process, however. Also the diagnoses given in the DSM-III are on the way to a unity of illness, which is laid out though the troubles at validation; their welcome descriptive neutrality cannot be retained. It was already believed possible to predict that the next version of the DSM would be nothing other than going from edition to edition of the Kraepelinian theory book, again appearing completely differently in idiopathic central areas.

Respect for the epochal achievement of Kraepelin should not stand in the way of a critical discussion on conceptions which eventually became clear that Kraepelin (18) expressed some doubts about. If the illness model is given up, it follows that one must hold specific known organic disturbances of different developments of illness as sometimes schizophrenia and sometimes affective disturbances; one does not come to psychopathological syndromes which could be enlarged by diagnoses in clinical use. Kraepelin's leading idea is presently remembered next to the consideration of developments of special expression criteria such as certain age limits, the changing expression of both idiopathic form areas and the unconnectedness of organic disorders. The biological model of illness is presently no longer used for the grounding of psychiatric systems, however it certifies usual thought patterns, which remained effective behind a pragmatic action of the setting up of diagnostic classification.

The projected meaning of certain neurotransmitters and receptors of effective psychopharmacology treatment for schizophrenic-like affective syndromes speaks for somatic deviation from norms but not for specific processes of illnesses. The disturbance of limbic and hypothalamic functions would speak for disturbances of impulses and affectivity which are characteristic for affective syndromes as restrictions or expansions of dynamics along with biorhythm disorders and which appear as an instability of dynamics in productive schizophrenic episodes. Here, we speak of a derailment of dynamics and in it we see the psychotic essence of idiopathic psychosyndromes as near to the target of somatic therapy. The dynamic derailment as an affective and reversible primary emotional disorder was seen before Kraepelin and could progress as secondary weaknesses. From the view of the Kraepelinic illness model this older concept taken from Griesinger was termed the theory of unity psychoses.

There are no sharp borders between affective and schizophrenic syndromes existing for a modified unity-psychosis summary of a derailment of dynamics. Above all affective disorders show overlaps on all sides if (in the majority) they are not comprised of a set phenomena such as madness or "tricking the senses". The schizophrenia - diagnosis primarily supports itself on a structural achievement of independence of set emerging phenomena of first rank symptoms. If the derailment of dynamic is clearly apparent behind these set phenomena (as occurs especially in acute psychotic episodes) and instability approaches a habitual phasic course with a manic influence, then symptoms can have many different meanings. The schizoaffective are in-between (16) in which psychopathological phenomena mix both forms, is indeed much bigger than we would like to admit in our efforts towards an exact boundary between affective and schizophrenic disorders.

Another problem which is similarly present with affective syndromes has to do with an entity of psychopathological phenomena through development criteria which is recognized as schizophrenic disorder with organic causes. It can also appear as a fundamentally organic occurrence somewhat like epilepsy or a misuse of certain drugs. Conventions which support themselves on the acceptance of several independent events of illness, forbid further talk on schizophrenia. However, these conventions are not compelling. It is possible that behind schizophrenic syndromes there are presumed somatic function disorders which are unspecified and which can arise from willingness just as much as from somatic occurrences of illness or can arise as a reaction to certain mental stressors. Even more important than somatic function disorders coming from different directions is the structure of personality from this viewpoint, which in similar ways answers in advance schizophrenic syndromes from a psychopathological viewpoint. The therapeutic pragmatic makes no differentiation here in any case: schizophrenic amphetamine psychoses or reactive psychoses are treated neuroleptically just as much as "genuine" schizophrenias.

From the viewpoint of the emerging illness model the schizophrenic disturbances in process are leading and originally seen as characteristic only for residual states of mind as the immediate result of a progressive illness of dementia praecox. In the meantime, doubt has been cast on the conception. Residual states of mind must also be included in the development of affective illnesses; it proves to be regressive in many ways; what remains as residue after the regression of productive stages of development is often nothing more than a bland dynamic insufficiency which was already set out in the weaknesses of the premorbid personality. Mundt's (21) monograph on the apathy syndromes of schizophrenics dealt with this connection. Much of what has become ascribed to the development of schizophrenic syndromes appears to first come out of the personality of the ill person. In the use of language, several structural dynamic conceptions asked what "derailment dynamic" is in a schizophrenic syndrome and which parts have a broken structural existence in the psychosis. It would have to be considered that structure and dynamics are narrowed together so that pathogenetic developments also must be summarized as structural-dynamic processes (13). Special to the interpretation of chronic developments the emphasis would be not on the derailment of biological functions but on the distortion of structure. If one holds to newer diagnostic categories the decision of chronicity of schizophrenic developments would fall on axis II of the DSM III.

As a development from early times which has been credited to Wing, Strauss, Carpenter and Bartko and which a whole issue of the *Schizophrenia Bulletin* was devoted to in 1985. The differentiation of positive and negative schizophrenic symptoms must be discussed. The differentiation can be traced back to Jackson and von Berrios and to Reynolds; all of them created simplifications with some plausibility. Crow (5) ordered positive symptoms as a (productive) type 1 and negative (deficient) type 2 (under the term dopamine-hypothesis) and Andreasen (1) developed a research tool for the detection of negative symptoms. English and American authors without knowledge of earlier discussions took up ideas which had belonged to German psychiatry since 1922. At the time Gruhle opposed von Berze's insufficiency hypothesis, that in many cases dementia praecox was a plus in impulses in the sense of a hyperfunction. Similarly the hypo- and hyper-phases of manic depressives according to Gruhle showed "some developments or phases of schizophrenia with a plus, some with a minus of mental activity". Through the gains of neuroleptic therapy Gruhle's differentiation has again become current, because it was not based on individual symptoms but rather the mental entirety. Some structure-dynamic beginnings (12) differentiated between a dynamic derailment of instability since 1959 which approach neuroleptics with their productive phenomena and one of a somatic therapy of hardly attainable dynamic insufficiency. G. Huber's shared research from 1957 (10) on brain atrophied changes and basic states and symptoms in schizophrenics remained unconsidered as Anglo-American authors began to concern themselves with similar questions. Huber's monograph (11) on the concept of a basic disorder avoided biases and critically opposed the difference between positive and negative schizophrenia.

In the long history of the concept of schizophrenia there were many wrong approaches taken but also many advances. Advances were primarily in the area of therapy and biological research with exact scientific methodology. To the special achievements of present-day psychiatry belongs the transformation of knowledge of gathered experiences into an empirical, verifiable knowledge of facts. The abundance of dates and detailed questions has become so big that connections often get lost. The author who fundamentally conceived the current question of schizophrenic vulnerability, under the direction of Zubin, was E. Kretschmer (19) who developed sensitive "insane-relations" which is already no longer valid. Empirical action relied on the operationalization of psychopathological phenomena, but did not yet lead to nosologically valid diagnostic differences. There are approaches to overcoming conventions of language barriers and school opinions as to what should be understood by schizophrenia. Up until now there is no clearly defined illness of "schizophrenia". The history of the concept of schizophrenia is in no way a history of medical discoveries. It is the history of the model of thought which psychiatry is oriented on.

References

1. Andreasen NC (1982) Negative Symptoms in schizophrenia. Arch Gen Psychiatry 39: 784-788

2. Berner P (1982) Psychiatrische Systematik. Huber, Bern Stuggart Wien

3. Berrios GE (1985) Positive and negative Symptoms and Jackson. Arch Gen Psychiatry 42: 95-97

4. Bleuler E (1908) Die Prognose der Dementia praecox (Schizophreniegruppe). Allg Z Psychiatr 65: 436-464

5. Crow TJ (1980) Molecular pathology of schizophrenia: More than one disease process? Br Med J 280: 66-68

6. Diagnostisches and Statistisches Manual psychischer Störungren DSM-III. Dt Bearb u Einf von Koehler K. Saß H (1984) Beltz, Weinheim Basel

7. Griesinger W (1861) Die Pathologie und Therapie der psychischen Krankheiten. Krabbe, Stuggart

8. Griesinger W (1868/69) Vortrag zur Eröffnung der psychiatrischen Klinik zu Berlin am 2. Mai 1867. Arch Psychiatr Nerevenkr 1: 143-158

9. Gruhle HW (1922) Die Psychologie der Dementia praecox. Z Gesamte Neurol Psychiatr 78: 454-471

10. Huber G (1957) Pneumencephalographische und psychopathologische Bilder bei endogenen Psychosen. Springer, Berlin Göttingen Heidelberg

11. Huber G (1986) In: Süllwold L, Huber G: Schizophrene Basisstörungen. Springer, Berlin Heidelberg New York Tokyo

12. Janzarik W (1959) Dynamische Grundkonstellationen in endogenen Psychosen. Springer, Berlin Göttingen Heidelberg

13. Janzarik W (1968) Schizophrene Verläufe. Springer, Berlin, Heidelberg New York

14. Janzarik W (1978) Wandlungen des Schizophreniebegriffes. Nervenarzt 49: 133-139

15. Janzarik W (1979) Die klinische Psychopathologie zwischen Griesinger und Kraepelin im Querschnitt des Jahres 1878. In: Janzarik W (Hrsg) Psychopathologie als Grundlagenwissenschaft. Enke, Stuttgart

16. Janzarik W (1980) Der schizoaffektive Zwischenbereich und die Lehre von den primären und sekundären Seelenstörungen. Nervenarzt 51: 272-279

17. Kraepelin E (1899) Psychiatrie. Barth, Leipzig

18. Kraepelin E (1920) Die Erscheinungsformen des Irreseins. Z Gesamte Neurol Psychiatr 62: 1-29

19. Kretschmer E (1966) Der sensitive Beziehungswahn. Springer, Berlin Heidelberg New York

20. Lange J (1922) Katatonische Erschinungen im Rahmen manischer Erkrankungen. Springer, Berlin

21. Mundt Chr (1985) Das Apathiesyndrom der Schizophrenen. Springer, Berlin Heidelberg New York

22. Pichot P (1983) Ein Jahrhundert Psychiatrie. Dacosta, Paris

23. Pope HG, Lipinski JF (1978) Diagnosis in schizophrenia and manic-depressive illness. Arch Gen Psychiatry 35: 811-828

24. Sander (1868/69) Über eine specielle Form der primären Verrücktheit. Arch Psychiatr Nervnekr 1: 387-419

25. Schneider K (1967) Klinische Psychopathologie. Thieme, Stuttgart

26. Schüle H (1878) Handbuch der Geisteskrankheiten. Vogel, Leipzig

27. Snell L (1865) Ueber Monomanie als primäre Form der Seelenstörung. Allg Z Psychiatr 22: 368-381

28. Westphal C (1878) Ueber die Verrücktheit. Allg Z Psychiatr 34: 252-257 (Ref)

29. Wilmanns K (1907) Zur Differentialdiagnostik der "funktionellen" Psychosen. Zentrealbl Nervenheilkd Psychiatr 30: 569-588

An Examination of the History of Concepts of Schizophrenia

Von C. Scharfetter

IN THE PREFACE of his famous monograph "Dementia Praecox, or Group of Schizophrenias", in 1911, Eugen Bleuler wrote:

> The whole idea of dementia praecox stems from Kraepelin. He is to be thanked for almost single-handedly creating an emphasis on grouping and detailing of particular symptoms.

Kraepelin developed the idea of dementia praecox from 1896 on.

What came before Kraepelin?

At the turning of the 19th century there were still no existing useful groupings of psychoses. Detailed descriptions and etiologic speculations were mixed in different attempts at classification. These, however, were unsatisfactory. Most effort on the subject was put into terminology, and there was an abundance of names for different manifestations of the appearance of insanity. However, the search for specific reasons and causes was without result; a pure descriptive, formal definition did not yet exist, nor, obviously did a psychopathological grouping of syndromes. Eventually, the idea of a unity of psychoses arose from Zeller and his student, Griesinger. Resulting clinical observations began to take a completely different course.

From the abundance of different manifestations and developments appearing in different cases, those with similar symptoms were searched out. In 1922, Bayle came up with the idea of progressive paralysis. A nosological unity was founded by him for the first time, with specific substratas and recognizable developments. From here, old psychiatric concepts (eg. melancholy, mania), could be changed into distinguishing signs of psychopathological conceptions of conditions. In overcoming old systems of classification of psychoses a procuration of the direction of the illness was strived for. The idea of a process of illness was created (H. Neumann, 1859). Neumann spoke of psychoses which left a permanent handicap. There were new criteria for classification: symptoms and developments led Falret (1851) to a definition of folie circulaire as an illness unity (Fischer). From this came the idea of unity psychosis.

Morel (1852, 1860) clearly expressed the problems involved in basing a classification of illness on causes, symptoms and developments. Morel first differentiated the term "démence praecox"; however, not because of indication of a unity of illness, but because of a patient, who after the age of 14, displayed hebephrenic symptoms in a process of "démence". Morel ranked dementia praecox with folie hereditaire. He was one of the first to link the meaning of hereditary disposition to the manifestations of psychoses.

Kahlbaum took psychiatry a step further (1863-1874) towards the current model, which is founded on clinical empiricism. After many problems and critical self-examination, he put forward his monograph on catatonia. He outlined a psychopathological concept; even our modern definition of easily recognizable signs such as waxy flexibility, jaw cramps, verbigeration (repetition of meaningless words), etc., can be traced back to him. He pointed to cyclical, changing developments and a relatively good remission ability. He also knew that certain catatonic psychoses could be life-threatening (the form which Stauder called "acute deathly catatonia"); v. Braunmühl called it "pernicious catatonia". The concept of hebephrenia already appeared in Kahlbaum's works; his descriptions are similar to those of Esquirol and Morel. Kahlbaum's student, Hecker, monographically depicted hebephrenia in 1871. He pointed to symptoms from puberty behavior, often defined with difficulty, often beginning chronically, and quickly leading to a clear dementia.

While catatonia and hebephrenia were seen as separate diseases to begin with, Fink (1881) spoke of a mixing of catatonic and hebephrenic symptoms , which attests that both these forms do, in fact, belong to one group.

In 1865, Snell described paranoid psychoses (monomanias) as a fundamental form of mental disorder close to melancholy and mania. (His descriptions are similar to Griesinger's "primary insanity".)

The principal of a classification of illnesses based on causes, symptoms, developments and expression soon led Kraepelin to an inclusion of previously predominantly clinically - symptomalogically defined concepts of catatonia and hebephrenia, and eventually led to the development of the concept of dementia praecox.

Emil Kraepelin already had much influence on the concepts of development and expression of mental diseases in the 1883 domain of psychiatry. In 1896 (in the 5th edition of his "Psychiatry") he included dementia praecox under the process of going insane (this corresponds to modern-day concepts of hebephrenia and dementia simplex), and dementia paranoia (which was not yet included as paranoid hallucinatoria or phantastica).

In 1889, (in the 6th edition), the term dementia praecox appeared as a larger concept in terminology of one of the two groups of functional (endogenous) psychoses. Kraepelin classified catatonia and hebephrenia as subgroups of dementia praecox (which further comprised dementia simplex) and dementia paranoia. Kraepelin himself knew that the term was not ideal: it was clear to him that dementia praecox had nothing to do with an intellectual or cognitive/memory weakness, but was fundamentally an affective "going insane." He also well knew that not all these psychoses began in youth, as praecox cases did, and that not all of them necessarily led to permanent declines.

In further editions (1903, 1909-1915), Kraepelin included dementia simplex in the subgroups; similarly the simple primary dementia, long recognized but little considered, was described in detail by Pick (1891) and Diem (1903). For Kraepelin, the basic characteristics among the manifold images and developments of dementia praecox were a loss of inner unity of thought, mind and performance of will.

In 1902, in the publication "Dementia Praecox" in the Journal of Mental Pathology (New York), Eugen Bleuler put forth a complete agreement with Kraepelin's concept of dementia praecox.

> My twenty year's experience has taught me to delineate the disease in the same manner as Kraepelin has done with the exception that I have not included the paranoid forms quite as extensively as the latter author has done. Now I think, however, that Kraepelin is right (p. 113).

In order to make a diagnosis, the grouping of illnesses according to symptoms and symptomatology must be sufficiently defined. Bleuler divided primary symptoms from secondary symptoms: the fundamental characteristics and essential symptoms of this psychosis are the breakdown of thought, including unfitting and incomprehensible behavior, and impaired intellectual, perceptive and memory functions. As Kraepelin knew, it deals with no ordinary dementia with alterations of intellectual and memory functions, but rather, with an emotional disturbance:

> The emotions are indifferent, inadequate, and not in conformity with the ideas of the patient's mind... such as alteration of the emotions in patients with an unimpaired consciousness and orientation is found in no other psychic affection. (p. 115).

Characteristic of this mental disturbance is a disturbance in association:

> That on the one hand the mental connections are interrupted here and there in an irregular manner, on the other hand, there appear thoughts, the connection of which with the preceding ones, either in part or as a whole, is not traceable. (p. 116)

Spontaneous speech can become incomprehensible (a "word salad", as Forel calls it). According to Bleuler, accidental accompanying symptoms are hallucinations, delusions and catatonic symptoms. Bleuler stressed that no definite borders were established between the subgroups, whose symptomologies overlapped in various ways.

Bleuler was also in agreement with Kraepelin that the illness did not have to begin in adolescence, and that it can be contained in any phase, where a development of "social healing" is possible. Whether or not this healing is scarless was uncertain. A defined pathological-anatomical or histological finding was not discovered.

Regarding the term "dementia praecox", Bleuler said:

> The term is not well-chosen; but the question is only that of a nomen et flatis vocis and not of the thing itself .(p. 120)

The ordering of symptoms into essential and accidental, the variability of age of contraction and differential developments and manifestations were all certain for Bleuler in 1902. In his further works, his descriptions of symptoms of dementia praecox remain as a disturbance in associations and affectivity; the disturbed behavior appears as autism (1908,1911). The basic differentiation of symptoms into primary and secondary remained a central concern. (1908, p. 454):

> Above all, we must strive for a differentiation between primary symptoms, which belong to the process of the disease and secondary, which are first developed through the reaction of the ill psyche to the influence of its surroundings.

The study of prognosis, because of outer, changing developments, allowed no division into subgroups (as Kraepelin also stressed in 1908, p. 447).

In 1908, Bleuler first suggested the term "schizophrenia" to replace the Kraepelinian terminology dementia praecox, and said "I believe that the rupture or fission of mental functions is a symptom of the entire group."

On this basis of terminology, Bleuler sought to grasp the (main) characteristic of this group of illnesses. The division into primary and secondary psychologically deprived symptoms and the question of a basic disturbance are closely connected with the name. "Schizophrenia" and the idea of a "disintegration psychosis" (Jahrmärker, 1908) were historically preparatory, as we will see.

The roots of the concept of psychic splitting go back to romantic thought patterns, and Herbarts psychology (1816) and theory of mental strengths which could ball together (complexes) and replace consciousness, as well as being able to dissociate. Esquirol (1838) already held this type of splitting of mental functions in many mental illnesses as true. H. Newmann (1859) saw a disintegration of consciousness through a loosening of mental connections in certain psychoses. Kahlbaum and his student Hecker maintained that described psychoses of hebephrenia and catatonia were not led by an intellectual and memory deterioration, but rather are characterized by an incongruency between comfortable mentality and the content of experience. In 1887, Neisser described the affective inaccessibility of many ill, and the non-correspondence of mental situations and the content of experience. In 1905, Neisser also talked of the disintegration of personality through dementia praecox.

Wernicke's (1880, 1894, 1896) sejunction hypothesis had become very well-known. With certain mental disorders, a loosening of structures of association occurs. He described schizophrenia (as we would say today), and maintained that "man is certainly comprised of a quantity of different personalities at the same time; we can show it's condition as a disintegration of individuality".

O. Gross (1904) took up Wernicke's hypothesis. He conveyed the automization of many catatonics as a secondary symptom coming from split off chains of association. He pointed to dissociative incoherence as characteristic of the disease, and proposed the name dementia sejunctiva for this psychosis. Janet (1889) and also Binet (1892) spoke of a mental dissociation and splitting as the result of a "general weakness of mental reality" (Griesinger p. 346), a "lowering of mental level" and a disturbance in the perception of reality. In this fashion, Masselon (1902, 1904) named the fundamental disintegration of dementia praecox a dissociation of mental functions. Bleuler (1902) mentions the splitting of mental functions. Stransky (1903, 1904, 1953) also mentioned the dissociation between feeling and intellect, the incongruency of thymo and noopsyche, the primary of dementia praecox, and suggested an indication of intrapsychic ataxia as a basic functional disorder. Those lacking a secure personality during puberty are disposed to such a process of dissociation. He also stressed that a disintegration in coordination did not have to be permanent.

Janet's idea of the "lowering of a mental level" was widespread, and was also suggested in Evensen's "ambly-noia" and in signs of hypophrenia which Berze (1903) suggested were characteristic of a basic disturbance of paranoia, and which later led him to see signs of central disintegration of dementia praecox as insufficient as leading to mental activity.

The ideas of mental and personality disintegration led to other suggestions for terminology based on the same considerations in the same year that Bleuler termed "schizophrenia". Wolff spoke of "dysphrenia", Zweig of "dementia dissecans", and Jahrmärker of "destruction psychosis". Through manifold considerations and searching for a name containing the essence of the disturbance, the way was prepared for Bleuler.

By 1918, Bleuler himself hailed the hypothesis of a disturbance in associations as an elementary symptom of schizophrenia; the disadvantages of the "embryonic condition of our psychology" (1911, preface) were already well-known.

Bleuler spoke of groups of schizophrenia, but not of a nosological unity. This should not be claimed in unknown etiology. The basic situations of illness is a "schizophrenic brain affection" (1911, p. 285), whose cause is unknown.

> Heredity plays a role in the etiology of schizophrenia. But it cannot be said how large or of what type its influence is. (1911, p. 285)

He saw mental causes as improbable: it comes from good anamesis:

> That mental experiences - naturally almost always of an agreeable nature - can produce schizophrenic symptoms. It is, however, highly unlikely that the disease is really brought out like this. Mental incidents trigger symptoms, but not the disease itself. (1911, p. 281)

This clear differentiation from pathogenetic and psychoreactive triggering factors was formulated by Bleuler in 1890 (p. 14/15):

> One differentiates two-fold causes: a disposition to the disease which lies dormant, and the opportunity cause, which brings the illness to expression. The greater the disposition for mental illness, the less effect opportunity causes may have.

With this, Bleuler prepared structural analyses of psychoses differing from pathogenetics and pathoplastics, later worked on by Birnbaum.

From occurring systematic psychoses similar to schizophrenia, Bleuler knew that there were also schizophrenic symptoms outside of this illness, which were summarized as schizophrenia.

> We know that chronic meningitis and brain traumas can show similar signs of illness to schizophrenia. (1911, p. 280)

Here we find thoughts that particular schizophrenic symptoms are not entirely specific to what we see as a union of symptoms of functional psychoses of schizophrenia. It was important to Kraepelin, and then Bleuler, that a diagnosis was not made on the grounds of several concepts of symptoms, but that an entire symptomological context had to be considered along with the living environment and body state.

Again Bleuler and the Zürich school are to thank for another meaningful development: the psychodynamic consideration. Bleuler and Freud's inclusions of psychoanalytic thoughts allows many symptoms to be seen through individual, personal reactions and life-destiny. Outside of biological considerations, with this came the psycho and sociogenetic point of view (now considered modern), of the problem of psychoreactive impulses and the importance of pathoplastics. In the recognition of psychological understanding, many symptoms of schizophrenia and phases of illness prepare a demand for a psychotherapy of schizophrenia.

I will briefly sketch the development of this theory:

In 1893, the joint work of Breuer and Freud on "the mental mechanisms of hysterical phenomena" was published. In 1894 and 1896, Freud tried to clarify the genesis of "schizophrenic" symptoms according to form and content of a patients life-history: the ego - incompatible is displaced and separated; this material leads to a complex image and reoccurs in a converted form. Psychosis is seen as a defense against this. In the same sense, Karl Abraham investigated the meaning of psychosexual traumas for dementia praecox (1907), and he contrasted it to hysteria (1908).

Bleuler in 1906-7, wrote on "Freudian Mechanisms in the Symptomatology of Psychoses". A great revelation for clinical psychiatry was the close application to the background of individual patients. This concern with the individual was new vis a vis the former predominant consideration of psychoses. In 1907, Jung published studies "On the Psychology of Dementia Praecox" from the Bleularian clinic. In these, he tried to establish the meaning of feeling - stressed complexes for the development of symptomology. At the time, Jung clearly stated

> on the question of etiology, that is to say, the essence of the question, one must stop (p. 43) The Freudian mechanisms do not suffice to explain why a dementia praecox develops, and not a hysteria. (p. 45)

Bleuler clearly says in "Causes of Complexes and Illnesses in Dementia Praecox" (1908) that primary symptoms of dementia praecox correspond to physical illness; however mental causes, affects, and complexes had further influences.

> The complexes are not the causes of illness, but rather opportunity causes for the formation of emerging symptoms and surely determined causes for the content of the latter... There is no person without complexes; the disease process also behaves in such a way.

So, with the endeavors of many, the concept of schizophrenia developed. In 1911, Bleuler left the question open as to whether schizophrenia was a unity of illnesses or not. Even today we do not know if it is a homogenous group.

Schizophrenia is still "quite nebulous" today (Kraepelin, 1903 p. 269). We have no specific etiology and pathogenesis or theory. The issue remains controversial.

Today, the clinical reality of doctors in its psychotic protégé should not be seen only as "Alienus mente"; the suffering of humans and a change in methodically fruitful research and therapy should be perceived. Kraepelin and Bleuler's concept is flexible and yet constant. It proves itself useful for many-sided research projects. It appears that Kraepelin and Bleuler knew the facts of the case.

References and Notes

1. General Historical Literature

Ackerknecht E.H.; Kurze Geschichte der Psychiatrie. Enke Stuttgart 1967. - Alexander F.G. und Selesnnick S.T.: Geschichte der Psychiatrie. Diana Zürich 1969.- Arndt E.: Über die Geschichte der Katatonie. Zbl. Nervenhk. 25, 81-121 (1902).- Birnbaum K.: Geschichte der psychiatrischen Wissenchaft. In: Hdb. der Geisteskrankheiten, hsg. v. O. Bumke, 1, allg. T. 1, 11-48 (1928).- Bleuler M.: Die Entwicklung der wissenschaftlichen Psychiatrie und medizinischen Psychologie in Zürich im vorigen halben Jahrhundert (1895-1945). Festschrift zur 200-Jahr-Feier der Naturforschenden Gesellschaft in Zürich (1746-1946). Zürich 1946.- Bleuler M.: Conceptions of schizophrenia within the last fifty years and today. Proc. Roy. Soc. Med. 56, 945-952 (1963).- Boor W. de: Psychiatrische Systematik. Springer Berlin-Göttingen-Heidelberg 1954.- Gruhle H.W.: Bleulers Schizophrenie und Kraepelins Dementia praecox. Zschr. Neurol. (Orig.) 17, 114-133 (1913).- Gruhle H.W.: Geschichtliches. In: Hdb. der Geisteskrankheiten, hsg. v. O. Bumke, 9, spez. T.V, 1-30 (1932).- Katzenstein R.: Karl Ludwig Kahlbaum und sein Beitrag zur Entwicklung der Psychiatrie. Diss. Zürich 1963.- Kirchhoff Th.: Geschichte der Psychiatrie. In: Handbuch der Psychiatrie, hsg. v. G. Aschaffenburg, Allg. T., 4. Abt. Deuticke Leipzig u. Wien 1912.- Kraepelin E.: Hundert Jahre Psychiatrie. Zschr. Neurol. 38, 161-275 (1918).- Pauleikhoff B.: Die Katatonie (1868-1968). Fortschr. Neurol. Psychiat. 37, 461-496 (1969).- Pethö B.:

Hundert Jahre Hebephrenie. Psychiatrie 24, 305-317 (1972).- Wyrsch J.: Zur Geschichte und Deutung der endogenen Psychosen. Thieme Stuttgart 1956.

2. Specific sources

Abraham K.: Über die Bedeutung sexueller Jugendtraumen fur die Symptomatologie der Dementia praecoxz. Zbl. Nervenhk. 30, (NF 18), 409-415 (1907).- Abraham K.: Die psychosexuellen Differenzen der Hysterie und der Dementia praecox. Zbl. Nervenhk. 31 (NF 19), 521-533 (1908).- Bayle A.L.J.: Recherches sur l'arachnitis chronique. Paris 1822.- Berze J.: Primärsymptom der Paranoia. Marhold Halle a.S. 1903.- Berze J.: Die primäre Insuffizienz der psychischen Aktivität; ihr Wesen, ihre Erscheinungen und ihre Bedeutung als Grundstörung der Dementia praecox und der Hypophrenie überhaupt. Deuticke Leipzig u. Wien 1914.- Binet A.: Les altérations de la personnalité. Paris 1892.- Bleuler E.: Die Behandlung der Geisteskranken im Privathaus. In: 15. Bericht des Zürcher Hülfsvereins für Geisteskranke, 13-31, Ulrich & Co. Zürich 1891.- Bleuler E.: Dementia praecox. J. Ment. Path. N.Y. 3, 113-120 (1902/1903).- Bleuler E.: Affektivität, Suggestibilität, Paranoia. Marhold Halle a.S. 1906. - Bleuler E.: Freudsche Mechanismen in der Symptomatologie von Psychosen. Psychiat. neurol. Wschr. 8, 316-318, 323-325, 338-340 (1906/1907).- Bleuler E.: Die Prognose der Dementia praecox (Schizophreniegruppe). Allg. Zschr. Psychiat. 65, 436-464 (1908). Bleuler E.: Komplexe und Krankheitsursachen bei Dementia praecox. Zbl. Nervenhk. 31, 220-227 (1908). Bleuler E.: Dementia praecox oder Gruppe der Schizophrenien. In: Handbuch der Psychiatrie, hsg. v. G. Aschaffenburg, Deuticke Leipzig u. Wien 1911.- Bleuler E.: Störung der Assoziationsspannung, ein Elementarsymptom der Schizophrenie. Eine Hypothese. Allg. Zschr. Psychiat. 74, 1-21 (1918).- Braunmühl A. von: Insulinschock und Heilkrampf in der Psychiatrie. 2. Aufl. Wissenschaftl. Verlagsanstalt Stuttgart 1947.- Breeuer J. und Freud S.: Über den psychischen Mechanismus hysterischer Phänomene. Neurol. Zbl. 12, 4-10 (1893).- Diem O.: Die einfache demente Form der Dementia praecox. Arch. Psychiat. 37, 111-187 (1903).- Esquirol J.E.D.: Des maladies mentales. Baillière Paris 1838.- Evensen: Die psychologische Grundlage... (1903), zit. nach E. Bleuler, 1911. Falret J.-P.- (Vorlesung am) Hospice de la Salpetrière. Gaz des Hop., 23. u. 24. Jahr, 1850 u. 1851.- Falret J-.P.: Leçons clinques de médecine mentale, faites à l'hospice de la Salptrière. Paris 1854. Falret J.-P.: Des maladies mentales et des asiles d'alienés Baillière Paris 1864. - Fink E.: Beitrag zur Kenntnis der Jugendirreseins. Allg. Zschr. Psychiat. 37, 490-520 (1881). Fischer-Homberger Esther: Das zirkuläre Irresein. Juris Druck Zürich 1968. - Forel A.: Die sexuelle Frage. E. Reinhardt München 1908.- Freud S.: Die Abwehrneuropsychosen. Neurol. Zbl. XIII, 362-364, 402-409 (1894).- Freud S.: Weitere Bemerkungen über Abwehrneuropsychosen. Neurol. Zbl. XV, 434-448 (1896).- Griesinger W.: Pathologie und Therapie der psychischen Krankheiten. Stuttgart 1845. - Gross O.: Über Bewußtseinszerfall. Mschr. Psychiat. 15, 45-51 (1904). - Hecker E.: Die Hebephrenie. Virchows Arch. path. Anat. 52, 394-429 (1871). - Herbart: Lehrbuch der Psychologie. Königsberg 1816.- Jahrmärker M.: Endzustände der Dementia praecox. Zbl. Nervenhk. 31 (NF 19), 489-497 (1908).- Janet P.: L'automatisme psychologique. Alcan Paris 1889. - Jaspers K.: Eifersuchtswahn. Zschr. Neurol. (Orig.) 1, 567-637 (1910).- Jaspers K.: Allgemeine Psychopathologie. 1. Aufl. Springer Berlin-Göttingen-Heidelberg 1913.- Jaspers K.: Kausale und verständliche Zusammenhänge zwischen Schicksal und Psychose bei der Dementia praecox (Schizophrenie).Zschr. Neurol. (Orig.) 14, 158-263 (1913). - Jung C.G.: Über die Psychologie der Dementia praecox. Marhold Halle a.S. 1907. Neudruck: Walter Olten u. Freiburg 1972. - Kahlbaum K.L.: Die Gruppierung der psychischen Krankheiten. Kafemann Danzig 1863. - Kahlbaum K.L.: Die Katationie oder das Spannungsirresein. Hirschwald Berlin 1874. - Kraepelin E.: Compendium der Psychiatrie. Abel Leipzig 1883. - Kraepelin E.: Psychiatrie. Ein Lehrbuch für Studierende und Ärzte. J.A. Barth Leipzig. 5. Ed. 1896, 6. Ed. 1899, 7. Ed. 1903, 8. Ed. 1909-1915. - Masselon R.: Psychologie des Déments précoces. Thèse de

Paris 1902. - Masselon R.: La Démence précoce. Joanin Paris 1904. - Meynert Th.: Psychiatrie. Klinik der Erkrankung des Vorderhirns. Braumüller Wien 1884. - Morel B.A.: Etudes cliniques: Traité théorique et pratique des Maladies Mentales. Masson Paris 1852-1853. - Morel B.A.: Traité des maladies mentales. Masson Paris 1860. - Neisser C.: Die Katatonie. Stuttgart 1887. - Neisser C.: Individualität und Psychose. Vortrag 1905, Berlin 1906 (zit. nach C.G. Jung). - Neumann H.: Lehrbuch der Psychiatrie. Enke Erlangen 1859. - Pick A.: Über primäre Demenz. Wandervorträge 1891. - Pinel Ph.: Traité médico-philosophique sur l'aliénation mentale, ou la manie. Richard, Caille et Ravier Paris 1801. - Snell: Über Monomanie als primäre Form der Seelenstörung. Allg. Z. Psychiat. 22, 368-381 (1865). - Stauder K.H.: Die tödliche Katatonie. Arch. Psychiat. 102, 614-634 (1934). - Stransky E.: Zur Kenntnis gewisser erworbener Blödsinnsformen (zugleich ein Beitrag zur Lehre von der Dementia praecox). Jb. Psychiat. Neurol. 24, 1-149 (1903). - Stransky E.: Zur Auffassung gewisser Symptome der Dementia praecox. Neurol. Zbl. 23, 1074-1085 (1904); 24, 1137-1143 (1904). - Stransky E.: Zur Lehre von der Dementia praecox. Zbl. Nervenhk. 27, 1-19 (1904). - Stransky E.: Von der Dementia praecox zur Schizophrenie. Schweiz. Arch. Neurol. 72, 319 bis 330 (1953). - Wernicke C.: Der wissenschaftliche Standpunkt in der Psychiatrie. Cassel 1880.- Wernicke C.: Grundriß der Psychiatrie. Thieme Leipzig 1 (1894), 2 (1896) (2. Aufl. 1900) .- Weygand W.: Alte Dementia praecox. Zbl. Nervenhk. 27 (NF 15), 613-625 (1904).- Wolff G.: Zur Frage der Benennung der Dementia praecox. Zbl. Nervenhk. 31 (NF 19), 856-858 (1908). - Zeller E.A.: Bericht über die Wirksamkeit der Heilanstalt Winnenthal von ihrer Eröffnung den 1. Maärz bis zum 28. Februar 1837. Med. Corr.bl. des Württemberg. ärztl. Vereins 7, 321. - Zweig A.: Dementia praecox jenseits des 30. Lebensjahres. Arch. Psychiat. 44, 1015-1035 (1908).

The Schizophrenic Defect

L. E. Bellomo

Summary: The author makes both a historical and up-to-date review of the "schizophrenic defect" concept (S.D.). He comes to the conclusion that this is the "morbid residual" or balance left as "ideo-affective" capital after every productive psychotic outbreak.

The S.D. is studied in a "medium and long term" ward with prevailing statistics amounting to 33% D.E. patients plus 9% active schizophrenic patients over a total average of 100 chronic hospitalized patients.

It was found out that 33% of the that universe had some scattered family whereas 19% of these patients had no family at all. The latter showed strong tendency towards isolation, slovenliness and "hospitalism". They became "passive-dependent" patients.

The situational framework is analyzed. Medical staff relationships with patients, type of treatment and the illusion created by "fictitious discharge" of D.E. under no favorable psycho-environmental conditions are taken into account.

Methods to improve the situation are then outlined and discussed. The following topics are considered: correct therapeutics, family therapy, sectorization, therapeutic community, transition homes, and current legislation.

"There is no one in the world more sensitive and more vulnerable to human acts than a schizophrenic" (Racamier).

History

SCHIZOPHRENIA HAS BEEN and continues being a terrible scourge, affecting from .8 to 1% of population. This means a percentage of 142 to 160 patients for every 100,000 people, which is particularly serious not only in the present, but also in remote periods.(23,43) In fact, in the Middle Ages, when the psychiatric nosology had not been established, schizophrenics traveled across Europe. However, we know that the order of the "Beguinas" (2) protected and gave them shelter in their convents.

The "beguinatos" represent some of the testimonies of psychiatric rehabilitation, creators of the hostels in the "half way houses" as they are called today. In the 19th century, Esquirol formed the first "home for the insane", and the mercenary Juan G. Jofre had founded in Valencia, in 1409, the first psychiatric hospital.(51)

The celebrity of Pinel (1745-1826), when he released the mentally sick in Bicetre, expanded scientific borders all over the world.(56)

The humanitarian policy of John Conolly (1794-1866), abolishing the methods of contention and punishment created the movement of non restraint.

In reality, it was observed that it did not work to open the confinement doors, if this strategy was not accompanied by humane therapy, a thesis supported by Sivaden.

With the industrial period, technical automatization of labour is added to the equation. And the chronic mentally sick falls into marginalization except for some actions of little risk that could be made by them.

This is how occupational therapy, recreation and expression work shops with application of specific techniques for mobilizations, resocialization and rehabilitation of the mentally ill, started.

Today, we have intra and extra hospital shops, called "sheltered", for the ill, whose labour activity stops being a competitive task to convert itself into a synergistic task with the therapy imposed by the medical team.

According to modern studies (23, 48), between 40 and 50% of chronic schizophrenic patients can return to the community free of symptoms produced for a period of 6 to 12 months and, from this percentage, some 75% to 80% of them finally relapse, as evolutive-processal and malignant forms of the disease.

Neurobiopathology

In general, the disease of schizophrenia evolves into the schizophrenic defect or residual form. However, recently in a scientific lecture by Crow and his colleagues (14) the conjecture is made of a probable molecular pathology in schizophrenic brains and the degree of sensibility in the dopaminergic receptors in the central nervous system; the dopaminergic hypersensitivity would open two different cases in the clinic and in the evolution of the illness:

a. The first, would be the consequence based in the lack of turn-over of the dopamine (DOPA), resistant psychopharmalogic response and accentuated productivity of the "negative" or deficiency symptoms, defect, affective blunting and poor vital impulse. The clinical forms simple and hebephrenia would be the most common in this area. The brain scanner would find ventricle dilation, and there would exist an insufficient response to the neuroleptics. That neurobiological profile would correspond to Crow's type II, and to the emotionally "froide" (cold or indifferent) described by Racamier.
b. The other form would be the Schneiderian type of schizophrenia, of the Heidelberg group (Mayer Gross, Jaspers and Gruhle); here, we would find too, the forms of chronic clinical paranoia and schizoaffective schizophrenia. These would correspond to the Crow type I, with a good response to the neuroleptics, great dopaminergic sensibility, with favorable prognosis, rapid remission of the symptomatology and defective evolution less rapid. For the great productivity of the symptoms, it would enter in the nomenclature as a form "hot" (chaude) of Racamier and Crow type I.

Because the type of possibilities of evolution of the disease, the road would be more frequent from type I to type II than from type II to type I, according to Crow. The evolution would depend, according to Mackay on the specific and individual sensibility of the dopaminergic receptors in the case of a prognosis or tendency of type II to type I, and reverse, from type I to type II (37).

Clinical

This chapter of psychiatry, constitutes one of the most complex, for this reason, many classic authors, such as Kraepelin, gave up finalizing the treatment for schizophrenia when it evolved to the defective form.

However, other focuses have come about from time to time. In fact, many modern and contemporary studies give us proof that from this morbid "residue" it is still possible to rescue undamaged parts of the patient's ego and work with them in an efficient way.

Schizophrenics, considered in generic way, do not dement. That concept was definitely finished by Bleuler (10) who discovered through large but productive analytical studies of schizophrenic scripts, although jargonophasic, inexplicable and misunderstandable, certain logic and meaning was hidden in their thinking.

This task continues for us even with the use of the psychopharmaceutical drugs and also so with the advent of the depot neuroleptics, group therapy, family, community and social support.

However, the first observations made by Kraepelin, Pinel, Esquirol and Morel, gave to the disease of schizophrenia the character of "dementia praecox" (1,10,32). Then, with the observations of Bleuler made in 1911 and 1913, it was shown that many schizophrenics did not evolve into a "dementia" condition, but surprised the observer with their lucidity, the recovery of their psychic functions in total and the magnificent connection that they established with reality in an altered way, validity came to the concept of "schizophrenic defect".

The French (19) gave it the name of "affaiblissement démentiel" (Verblödung, from the German); defining a deficit (defekt) to the nosology connected to the Bleulerian pseudodemential form or type (19,45).

To the "process" of destruction of the psyche, of the inauguration of the affective-volitive emptiness, of the "vital loss with reality": such as Minkowski affirmed and the irremediable descent into the vacuum "cold and glacial emotion secures pseudo-legitimacy within a conduct illogical and irrational - the affective indifference" (40), is added to the intellectual decline, the loss of the preventive values, the incoherent message, absurd, without direction or sense. illogical and irrational.

After the new significance of the world and the "revelation" had ceased, there remained the defect, as Conrad says, which would be the residual of the conceptual main disorder is retained as a consequence and after the episode, a schizophrenic shoot (as of a plant), the consecutive "footprint of the disease" of the productive preceding phase (5,15).

For the psychiatry of Schneider, Mayer Gross and Jaspers, the appearance of primary symptoms, major and pathognomic of schizophrenia are equivalent to an organic disorder. Jaspers absorbs the new significance and he breaks the life line of the personality, without psychocorrective concomitants that justify it, or determining psychotraumatic affectives important for the appearance of the "shoot", as a result of an organic process whose etiopathogenial cause is still obscure (41,50).

The break of the biographic life line of the individual would be the pathogenic result of that disorder; the theme picked as a final vector for the psychotic, and deliriant associations would be the pathoplastic of schizophrenia, generally associated with "paranoia delirium of influence", whose relation is self-referential and prejudiced (19).

Every "shoot" follows a residual and defective state every time more serious and clinically worse than the patient's previous state.

The ill person is not productive as he is in the decisive period or with the psychotic "positive" emergents from the subcortical subconscious liberation of the personality, of the "psychic disintegration" and the break up of the ego, as H. Ey wrote (19).

In the shoot's term, the DSM III postulates the primary symptoms of schizophrenia; then describes the symptoms of the "defect" (16).

The residual phase is predominated by the negative symptoms or deficits of H. Ey. There persists the isolation, collapse of the cognitive sphere, extravagant conduct, the deficit of cleanliness and the danger of impulsive or explosive acts. The affect remains blunted and flat with vague language, disintegrated, without sense or precision. The ideation is full of absurd and strange ideas, with abundant emphasis placed on the incoherent messages, the clairvoyance, the telepathic powers, the "sixth sense" and the autoreferential ideas (9,18,41,58). The Wechsler scale shows a percentage of deterioration that is always greater than 27 or 30%.

The World Health Organization (WHO) has remarked that the primary symptoms of the "schizophrenic defect", and the criteria of DSM III and WHO (42) are very similar. The characteristic of the "defect" is the impulse's weakness of the global energetic activity and the lack of "vigourous life" that Federn and Weiss called feeling's absence of the "ego's catexia"(22,57). The presence of the affective bluntness is accompanied by strange disorders in the corporal sphere; the alterations of the somatic area imitate the psychotic perturbations of the hypochondriac delirium. For example, the ill person believes, with delirious conviction, to have blocked a bronchus, "that from the stomach they call him, because the brain's radar is broken"...

We have observed that all these troubles are presented as complaints, with a mix of indignation and amazement and formulated interrogatively, e.g.: How is it possible that they use me when I am sleeping?! Why do they abuse me sucking my blood?!... These questions impress the observer counter transferentially, because they are statements without answer.

The ill person or (patient) is abandoned and falls in to the most dark hospital dependency. They beg for a penny or a cigarette, they ask the time, perhaps to know if it is time to eat; they are found collecting garbage, old clothes, and other useless goods.

They are the sick that scare those that visit the large asylums, for the first time, causing a strong feeling of therapeutic impotence.

The weight loss, associated with the bulimia is very common as it is TBC in the leptosomic "defect"(39). Diabetes is frequent in the "picnicker", and the appearance of convulsions is a potential, without epileptic antecedents and with E.E.G. normal.

Treatment

Individually, in dealing with the disease, there is no other alternative than instituting a "therapeutic synergy" which combines the biological therapy, psychopharmacologic, individual psychotherapeutic, communicative and psychosocial groups(4).

In general, we can say that the treatment should be constructed on:

1. Attendance of a medical team.
2. Maintenance of the neuropsychopharmologic therapy.
3. Maintenance of psychological setting contingency with family, social and community all a part of rehabilitation.

Medical attendance (medication, habits, life style): The therapist will be the one who responds to questions of the patient and his family, converting himself into a "messenger of reality"(19,46).

For some years now, the depot neuroleptics have been adding themselves to the oral ingestion of the incisive antipsychotic psychopharmacist, causing a reduction of the habitual doses of the latter, with the corresponding advantages, which is secure and supervised administration, to get a correct plasma level in the blood of neuroleptics sufficiently stable and efficient to get the doses of maintenance and quell the psychotic crisis, to keep the ill connected to reality. These anti-psychotics function as antihallucinolitics, antideliriants and antiautistics (12,33,34).

With respect to the style and habits of life recommended, we will try to link the feeling of the "necessity of working to be able to eat" and to relate this effective labour therapy with daily meals. The lack of supervision in such aspect would bring undoubtedly, a decline and a deterioration of the conduct and self-esteem of the patient, who is abandoned autisticly to his fantasies (44).

Individual psychotherapy. Family and psychosocial environment of the schizophrenic

Individual psychotherapy: From a psychotherapeutic point of view, the benefits of orthodox psychoanalysis, applied to schizophrenics are increasingly scarce(4). Freud did not accept the application of this technique in the "narcissistic neurosis" (psychosis sch.), for the great difficulty in transfer and for what Jung called the "introversion of the libido"(21).

However, analysts such as Searles (52), Sechehaye (51), Frieda Fromm-Reichmann (47), Nach and others, have proposed changes to the analytic classical technique, conjecturing that the schizophrenic has a rudimentary and precarious ability to establish "object relations" with the analyst, being possible to develop a psychotic transference.

Family: With respect to the family, all studies in the beginning focused their attention on the "schizophrenic mother", with emphasis on a type of mother who lacks capacity for enjoyment.

The works of Anna Freud, Spitz and Margaret Mahler talk about a type of mother who does not permit close attachment with her child.

Emotionally cold, distant, perfectionist, restrictive, voluble, intrusive and incapable of giving and receiving affection, it is as though a definition has been made in a wide and generic way.

Also the schizophrenic's father is an indistinct figure, without precise limits and non-participating. "Managed as a puppet by his wife" as Ramon Melgar (38) affirms: fails even to pretend to assume his legislative functions, control and order. The schizophrenic's family act as Pichon Rivière expresses it, as a uniform set of individualities that try to isolate him, put him away from the family, treating him as the "sacrificial goat" of a set of abnormalities that are kept latent and hidden within the family.

From my experience, I can say that the schizophrenic is unwanted by the family and is put away (6).

Lately, Nina Schooler has successfully proposed the instructive pedagogical family psychotherapy of the schizophrenic combined with chemotherapy.

Rehabilitation

Causation: A study (7) investigating prevalence statistics of the residual schizophrenia (WHO, 295.6), concluded that there is a family tendency to abandon the patient to the hospital in an open as well as a suspicious way.

In 100 patients, who were between 18 and 75 years old, 33% with diagnosis of "schizophrenic defect"; 9% were active schizophrenics; with a global total of 42%.

81% had a nuclear family; 50% were visited with regularity; 9% with no family at all, these days designated as "passive dependent", which happens to be strong index of social isolation, hospitalism and abandonment.

With respect to the 33% of "defect patients", 81.8% had a dispersed family; and 18.2% no family at all, repeating a similar proportion of patient in the general sample, in a similar manner.

Now, in the 42 female schizophrenics (33 residuals and 9 active) 17 of them have a chronic state (chronic hospitalization); 10 of the patients were leaders of the tasks in the pavilion; they kept a balance in the execution of the personal tasks such as: messages, co-operation with the rest, etc..., two of them were incapable and the rest, the 13% attended the sheltered shops in and outside of the hospital, CONET and the Club of Recreation.

Full Situation: We observed that in the sample of 33% of defective patients who had a family link, they took the patient home with them.

When we talk about releasing patients from the hospital we mean "release with dignity" and that implies medical responsibilities shared with the family (17).

Required is: a. Improvement in the mental state of the patient; b. Family or stable substitute; c. Ambulatory consultation with medical and psychotherapeutic follow up; d. A proper legal and regularized situation, such as the possibility to develop labor tasks intra or extrahospital work in shops, Day Hospital, CONET (National Council of Technical Education), etc .

The statistical proof and evaluation made us think that the family with a strong connection to the pathology, can co-operate as an additional therapeutic aid, but cannot take full care.

Since 1955 the USA has implemented numerous Centres for Mental Health, which was ratified by J.F. Kennedy on May 2, 1963.

Ten years later: skepticism. R. Reich, expressed that it was "cruel, hostile, even inhuman" to leave mental incapables in the community(31).

What happened?... The psychiatrist treated ambulatorily in the centres for health and had high numbers of discharges, but also the number of re-admissions was high, and came from lack of psychoambiental support, a phenomenon that Efrain Gómez called "the revolving door"(20). In reality, that discharges were "high" was fictitious, counting a success of the sanitary policy, but really false without taking into consideration all facts of risk as a truth.

From the stable patients (22-34%) arise the "leaders" of the community of patients who offer support in personal, group and community form, where they are responsible for serious situations of emergency (eg. power cuts, sudden death, etc.).

For being the most lucid, they also communicate with doctors and personnel. Sometimes the information to the chief is distorted, because they expect to get a punishment from a nurse, and in that way compensate certain resentments.

Erving Goffman (26), brings these facts as signs of "suffering of the ego" in an institution, eg. bad food, overcrowding, juridicial disidentification, etc.

The defective and indigent patient asks for unachievable improvements and when he has them, he does not know what to do with them (1,11,28).

Maxwell Jones insists that when the patient does not find the answers to his questions immediately, then he goes back to the community of sick people to look for the answers.

Undoubtedly a deficient personnel which does not know, or is incapable of distinguishing a deliriant idea, is exposed to the mercy of the psychopathic management of the sick (30).

In the asylum, there is a very strange phenomena that has occurred, from the most absolute permissibility to an extreme repression, similar to those in the concentration camp.

The patient is addicted to intrigues and uses them as techniques "of management" or seduction, pretending a semiadaptation or a fake "clinical improvement".

The personnel work with a pessimistic reality. Most of the time doctors do not tolerate madness, they feel a great deal of guilt, when they do not succeed in their task.

It used to happen that they project their persecutory anxieties on to the authorities of the institution, falling into a quasifeudal isolation in their services, or they are seduced by the elaboration of antipsychiatric ideas.

It has to be added that the role of irresponsible media dramatizing, makes the situation sadder and more difficult (6).

How to correct this picture? Schizophrenia is a clinical entity defined. These are medical-psychiatric problems that cannot be ignored, nor disqualified.

The famous Baruk insisted with acute observation that the mentally ill, no matter how crazy he is, he never loses his sense of justice, honesty, goodness and professional authority (53). Pinel affirmed that the leader most respected by the insane was the one, who knew how to inspire respect from his authority, not abusing it (49). Sometimes more is made from the conduct and the example than from therapy.

After what we just said, we could affirm with the School of Rapaport, Kris and Loewstein, that the schizophrenic patient has areas "free of conflict" that have not been significantly damaged and with them it is possible to try rehabilitation (29). One needs to add good treatment, responsible medical attention, and structured counseling.

Therapeutic community: The therapeutic community of Maxwell Jones looks for the readaptation of the schizophrenic defect. Implemented as a systematic methodology, with all personnel and patients, a. Democratic problem solving; b. Incentive reciprocity in the comprehension of individual problems; c. Moderation of intrigues, twisted versions of reality as "leaders" used to do to gain some privileges; and d. Revaluation of solidarity within the "passive-dependent" group.

Besides, future projects are discussed and evaluated to see if the messages have been received by the rest of the patients. To rescue the most sane, to reaffirm the criteria of reality of the rest.

The complaints of the psychotics, sometimes are important to solve difficulties. To satisfy them there is a lack of gratitude, that is reflected as a countertransferential feeling of impotence and of indignation for the lack of recognition for the effort.

That is why the role of the community is to force the patient to leave the level of passivity. The obligation to participate and to express is fundamental, so the recognition to avoid delirium, deficit and passivity.

Shops - "Homes of transition" Legislation: All types of therapy to mobilize the patient in his corporal and physical expression are beneficial. In that sense, the shops have good results.

To use expressive techniques in accordance with the patient's self-defenses, is successful. For example, a female patient with obsessive defenses will do better in tasks of ceramics or binding; the anxious more suited in kitchen tasks; other with artistic qualities of sublimation will use painting. * (*We must mention and recognize the work done in Argentina by our friend, Dr. Eugenio López Gómara, a prestigious psychiatrist and aesthete, who made possible when working for the Borda Hospital, one of the shops (Talleres) of "plastic expression" for mental patients, best equipped, and which has given us precious artistic testimonies, today, famous internationally among the students of the difficult world of the psychopathologic art.)

The same criterion is applied for the extrahospital shops (Talleres) in all national borders (44).

The patient should be "stimulated and required, not only by the psychiatric personnel, but also by his fellows, to assume and feel realizing a productive task, inserted into the hospital, social of labour life" (54 op. cit. 133).

Another preventive measure has been the "hostels of transition" or half way houses, in our environment successfully employed by Dr. Catalina Gimeno, as a target on this new community task (24,25).

It is about homes, where the chronic psychotic patient has been selected for the low level of psychotic productivity, with areas of the ego free of conflicts and useful, levels of self and controllable heteroimpulsivity, with familiar selective isolation and with a certain degree of lucidity to contact with other chronic patients.

In the hostels he may live with a security margin and supported by the technical supervisor or specialized "conductor guide", who controls his medication and his condition of life.

These houses or homes are donated by the community; patients realize tasks in common, help, cook or organize labour tasks, entertainment and sane and constructive pastimes.

These creative tasks and of life together can be paid or unpaid. The schizophrenic's concern about money is relatively small, if he has food, cigarettes, etc. In Argentina, Dr. Domingo Cabred (1859-1929), established the "peculio" for the sick, dignifying the ill person in the (Open Door) Hospital, abolishing the arbitrary contention and the authoritarianism.

The legislation has also advanced with the Law 22431 or "Law of integral protection system to the Handicapped persons", and the Law 22914 or "Law of protection for the mentally ill".

The residual schizophrenic is a sick person refractory enough to leave his weakness, apathy and selfism; it is necessary, therefore, to create in the patient - during his rehabilitation - the feeling to relate the work with daily food, creating a "feeling to relate the work with daily food", creating a "feeling of necessity", to connect the obligation to the gratification.

What is the result without the inertia and the therapeutic apathy produced by the skepticism about cure? As Maxwell Jones would respond: the result will be that the sick looks for his own interrogating the patients, dictated by his hallucinations and delirium, within the sick intrahospital community, falls into the most absurd and abject hospitalism.

The hospital will be his tomb, death will be the fantasy, primary savior and rescuer, and the doctor, acting to his therapeutic shame and against his Hippocratic oath - the scientific gravedigger in the eyes of history.❧

References

1. Arieti, S. - Interpretation of Schizophrenia. New York. Brunner, 1955.

2. Auger, Chanoine A. Les Béguinages, 1906. En: Biblioteca Colegio Máximo San Miguel (BA), Ubic. 30919.

3. Bateson, G. y cols. - Interacci—n Familiar, Buenos Aires, Tiempo contemporáneo, 1971.

4. Bellak, L. - Esquizofrenia p: 417-535, Barcelona, Herder, 1962.

5. Bellomo, L. E. - El per'odo de incubaci—n en la psicosis. Rev Neuro-Psiquiát (Argentina) 1980, 11, 1-96 (1).

6. Bellomo, L.E. - La réinsertion sociale de l'aliéné, surtout du schizophrène chronique rèsiduel- Un problème de prévention terciaire au sujet de la santé mentale. Grenoble, XIXème Congres de la UNAFAM, X, 1986.

7. Bellomo, L.E. y cols - Prevalencia estadística de la esquizofrenia residual (OMS 259.6) en una Sala de Mediano y Largo Plazo, Buenos Aires, Jornadas Científicas del Hospital Nacional Dr. Braulio Moyano, 1985.

8. Bion, W.R. - Aprendiendo de la experiencia. Buenos Aires, Paidós, 1966.

9. Bumke, O. - Nuevo Tratado de Enfermedades Mentales p: 733-736, Seix Editor, 1946.

10. Bleuler, E. - Demencia Precoz- El grupo de las esquzofrenias Ed. Hormé, Buenos Aires, Paidós, 1960.

11. Caudill, W. - El Hospital Psiquiátrico como Comunidad Terapéutica, Buenos Aires, Ed. Escuela, 1966.

12. Colonna, L.; Petit, M.; Dollfus, S. - Neuroleptiques. En Encyc Méd Quir Psychiat (EMQ, Psy) Paris 37860 B10-1-1986.

13. Caplan, G. - Principios de Psiquiatriá Preventiva. Buenos Aires, Paidós, 1980.

14. Crow, T.J. - Molecular pathology of schizophrenia: more than one disease process. Brit Med J, 1980, 6207, 66-68.

15. Conrad, K. - La esquizofrenia incipiente. Barcelona, Labor, 1955.

16. (DSM-III), México, Masson, 1984.

17. Duarte, A. - Rehabilitación del paciente psicótico crónico, Buenos Aires, Jornadas de la Asociación Argentina de Psiquiatras, Academia Nacional de Medicina, 1979.

18. Detre, P. y Jarecki, H. - Terapéutica Psiquiátrica. Salvat, 1974.

19. Ey, H. - Formes évolutives, rémissions. formes terminales. Problèmes du pronostic des schizophrénies. En EMQ Psy, Paris. 35285 A10-1972.

20. Gomez, E.A. - El problema del enfermo mental crónico indigente. Acta psiquiát psicol Amér lat, 1983, 29, 213-222.

21. Freud, S. - Sobre los tipos de adquisición de la neurosis, p: 978-981 T. 1 Obras completas, Madrid, Biblioteca Nueva, 1948.

22. Federn, P. - Ego Psychology and the Psychoses. New York, Baar Books, 1952. (Hay versión castellana: Amorrortu).

23. Freedman, A. and Kaplan, H. - Comprehensive Textbook of Psychiatry, Baltimore, 1967.

24. Gimeno, C. - Relato de una experiencia de tres anos en la organización de un hostal extrahospitalario, Buenos Aires, Jornadas Cientificas del Hospital Nacional Dr. Braulio Moyano, 1985.

25. Gimeno, C. - Diversas modalidades de instituciones posthospitalarias de transición, casas de mitad de camino, familias sustitutas, aldeas de pacientes, Buenos Aires, Jornadas Científicas del Lospital Nacional Dr. Braulio Moyano, 1985.

26. Goffman, E. - Internados p: 65-109, 103-173, 2da. ed. Buenos Aires, Amorrortu, 1972.

27. Goldember, M. - Programa Nacional de Salud Mental, DNSM, 1984.

28. Gralnik, A. - El hospital psiquiátrico como instrumento terapéutico. Buenos Aires, Paidós, 1984.

29. Hartman, H.; Kris, E.; Lowenstein, R.M. - Comments on the formation of Psychic Structure. En The Psychological Study of the Child 2 p: 11-38. New York, International Universities Press, 1946.

30. Jones, M. - The concept of Therapeutic Community. Am J. Psych, 7, 647- 650, 1956.

31. Jones, N. - Psiquiatría social. Buenos Aires, Ed. Escuela, 1962.

32. Kreaepelin, E. - Psychiatrie-Dementia Praecox p: 668-972. Leipzig, Johan Ambrosius Barth Edt., 1913.

33. Lambert, P.A.; Guyotat, J. - Neuroleptiques à action prolongée. En EMQ Psy, Paris 378060 B 40-10-1972.

34. Lipton, M.A.; Di Mascio, A,; Killan, K. - Psychopharmacology: a Generation of Progress. New York, Raven Press, 1978. (Hay versión castellana).

35. Loudet, O; Loudet, O.E. - Historia de la Psiquiatría Argentina Buenos Aires, Troquel, 1971.

36. Mahler, M. y cols. - El nacimiento psicológico del infante humano Ed. Cosin-Lumen, 1977.

37. Mackay, A.V.P. - Positivity of Schizophrenic Symptoms and the Role of Dopamine. Brit J Psyc, 1980, 137, 379-386..

38. Melgar, R. - Familia y esquizofrenia. Neuropsiquiat 1975, Ano VI, Nro. 2, 3 IV-IX.

39. Melgar, R. - Tuberculosis y Psicopatiás. Especial referencia a esa presunta etiologiá en las psicosis discordantes, 1937. Tesis doctoral. Faculated de Medicina, Universidad de Buenoes Aires, Ubic 4457.

40. Minkowski, E. - La esquizofreniaq. Psicopatología de los esquizoides y de los esquizofrénicos. Buenos Aires, Paidós, 1960.

41. Mayer-Gross, W.; Slater, E.; Roth, M. - Psiquiatría Clínica T.I. p: 399 y sig. Buenos Aires, Paidós, 1974.

42. Organizacion Mundial De La Salud (OMS) - Lista tabular DNSM de la Dirección Nacional de Salud Mental OSM 295.6. Restzustand esquizofrenico p: 16. Buenos Aires, 1980.

43. Pages Larraya F. y cols. - Prevalencia institucional de la Patología Mental en la República Argentina. Documenta Laboris, PEPSI, CONICET IV, 13, Buenos Aires, 1981.

44. Phillpot, E.; Iroz, J.C. y cols. - La rehabilitación del esquizofrénico en los Talleres Nacionales Protegidos, Azul, Primeras Jornadas de Psiquiatría Institucional, 1983.

45. Peron-Magnan, P. - Chimiothérapie et évolution des schizophrenies Conf Psychiat, 1968, 12, 125-137.

46. Racamier, P.C. - L'interprétation psychanalytique des schizophrénies 1957 Evol Psychiat, 79, 47-91 y en EMQ Psy, Paris, 37291 A-10-1976.

47. Reichman, F. - Psicoterapia en las psicosis, Ed. Hormé, Buenos Aires, Paidós, 1962.

48. Salomon, P.; Patch, V. - Manualde Psiquiatría p: 105-115. México, El Manual Moderno, 1972.

49. Semelaigne, R. - Les grands aliénistes français- Pinel, Ph. p: 109. Paris, Ed. Steinhed, 1894.

'50. Schneider, K. - Patopsicología Clinica p: 191 y sig. Madrid. Paz Montalvo, 1963.

51. Sechehaye, M.A. - La realización simbólica. México, Fondo de Cultura Económica, 1950.

52. Searles, H. - Escritos sobre esquizofrenia p: 69-106 y 165-208. Barcelona, Gedisa, 1980.

53. Sauri, J.J. - Historia de las Ideas Psiquiátricas (Pinel) p: 392-404. Buenos Aires, Carlos Lohlé, 1969.

54. Sivadon, P. - Psychopathologie du travail Evol Psychiat, 1952, 3, 451-474.

55. Schooler, N. - The Efficacy of Antipsychotic drugs and Family Therapy in Maintenance Treatments of Schizophrenia. J. Clin Psychopharm, 6 ii 1-19 s.

56. Vidart, L. y Juglard, J. - A propos de l'action de Philippe Pinel à l'Hospice de Bicetre. Ann Méd-Psychol, 1976, 2, 55-59.

57. Weiss, E.- Los fundamentos de la psicodinámica. Psique, 1957.

58. Wyrsch, J. - Esquizofrenia. En: Reichardt M. Psiquiatr'a General y Especial, p: 345-395. Madrid, Gredos, 1955.

59. Zilboorg, G. y Henry, G. - Historia de la Psicolog'a Medica p: 499-506-637. Buenos Aires, Hachette, 1945.

The History of the Treatment of the Indigent Chronic Mental Patient

E. Gomez

Summary: The history of the treatment of the severely chronic mentally ill since Pinel and the French Revolution is reviewed in order to demonstrate that a persistent and cyclical pattern of neglect followed by periods of protest and reform, has characterized the treatment and management of the chronic patient. The roots of the pattern of neglect are many, to understand them a historical and psychodynamic approach is necessary. The roots of neglect are found to be in the patients themselves, the therapists, society and the methods of treatment. The review of the literature and pertinent research reveal fragmentation and incoherencies reminiscent of the psychiatric illness itself. An integrated biopsychosocial approach which would give clinical coherence and some conceptual clarity is suggested to facilitate clinical work and more research.

"THE COMBINATION of causes to explain any phenomenon in particular, is beyond the human intelligence. But the will to look for these causes is natural in man. Sometimes, without considering the variety and complexity of the conditions, any of those causes in separate forms seem to be the cause, because man always picks the first approximation. So, man says: here is the cause" (29). This quotation taken from: *War and Peace"* where Tolstoy talks about causes of the Napoleonic wars, explaining the defeat of not only the army, but also of the French people. In a certain way the same quotation is useful to explain causes of a mental illness such as schizophrenia, as external and internal wars and perhaps a single defeat. The reference can also be applied to Harvard's Lazare's suggestion about psychiatry, in general and schizophrenia, in particular (19). He thinks that current psychiatry depends on 4 models, which are in theory, radically different from one another but in practice, they are complementary.

Lazare gives the example of a schizophrenic patient, who receives psychotherapy in both individual and in group format.

It uses, the method of pride and punishment to modify conduct, so he demonstrates that we continue doing what Hippocrates did in this time. Nobody has been capable enough to put together, in a common language the contents of the modern psychiatry.

Engel has tried to respond to this need with bio-psycho-social models (7) to overcome the method used by Plato and Aristotle, expanding the method of biomedicine, that attempts to reduce everything to a factorial analysis of physical-chemical reactions.

Psychology and sociology have tried to explain the human experience using generalities and abstractions based on statistics. What we need is a model which is clinically coherent and consistent, flexible enough to be modified when required. the bio-psycho-social model focuses on interactions of biological, psychological and social processes using the theory of systems.

Another problem of great consequence has been the lack of definite criteria for diagnosis of mental disorders. Clinicians and investigators from different countries do not have a common language with which to communicate. Fortunately, the Research Diagnostic Criteria and DSM III in USA and the International Classification of Illness, 9th edition in other countries, will bring better results in the future.

One of the reasons to pay more attention to diagnosis is the increase of psychiatric incapability in those countries called consumers because of: methods of payment, facility of compensation, and bureaucracy. It is to be noted that in consumer societies, it is more important to be a consumer than a contributor.

History

There are three periods which may be considered as "natural experiments", they reveal the conditions under which the psychiatric incapabilities are produced or recuperative processes facilitated.

These experiments were not planned and they took place: a) beginning of 19th century, b) 100 years later and c) after the Second World War. Before Pinel and the French Revolution, the mental patient was confined to dungeons together with criminals, chained and exposed to the public for money (32).

Pinel observed that the conduct of these unfortunates was a consequence not of having the sickness but of being treated like that. Convinced of the rightness of this hypothesis, Pinel decided to release some patients in Bicetre and the first patient released, rather than attack him, knelt down and kissed his feet.

Almost at the same time, alienists in other countries of Europe, were observing the same phenomenon and having the same experiences. All this started a new treatment called Moral Treatment. Under the influence of this more humane form of treating the alienated, the breakdown of personality and incapacity diminished in a spectacular way.

In the middle of 19th century, under influence of Quakerism in England, asylums were converted to open form. With emphasis the treatment concentrated on freedom, persuasion, rational communication and normal interpersonal interaction.

Not only doctors, but also relatives, contributed to cure the patients. The "indices of cure" got up to 100%. However, apparently in following days relapse was frequent.

Just a little before the 20th century, with the Industrial Revolution and the discovery of the Treponema Pallidum - cause of general progressive paralysis - interest in moral treatment waned and, without interpersonal relations, the index of cure dropped considerably.

Mental patients started to go to mental hospitals, which originated a perpetual imprisonment. Because of the demographic explosion, these kinds of mental institutions were converted into a storage of human waste. The emphasis on etiologic factors and organic treatments, was reflected in that Wagner-Jauregg and Egaz Moniz won the Nobel Prize. The first for treating the neurosyphilis with artificial fever and the second for introducing neurosurgical techniques. Freud, however, only received a literature prize.

Exceptions to the rule of abandonment and neglect were the work of Kraepelin whose Treatise in Psychiatry went through 9 editions. Kraepelin separated the dementia praecox from the manic depressive psychosis. Based in the natural history of the illness observed that the dementia praecox deteriorated but not the depressive psychosis. So, the problem was that in order to get a definite diagnosis a wait of many years was required until deterioration appeared (17).

Bleuler tried to solve this impasse in his book: Dementia Praecox or The Group of Schizophrenias, written in German in 1911, translated into English in 1950. He suggests that "not all schizophrenias deteriorate" and he adds: "some schizophrenics do not even go to see the psychiatrist" (1). Freud on the other hand, compared the psychosis with dreams, described two levels of intellectual function, differentiated the defensive neurotic mechanisms from psychotics, pointed out the regressive characteristic of the schizophrenic process and also the restitutive mechanisms of the illness.

His contribution was more important because of his ideas on the symbolic significance of psychotic symptoms rather than just a simple description of the phenomena (9). It is really unfortunate that Freud did not continue writing about psychosis after 1926, when he revised drastically his original theory about anguish.

Jung, Bleuler's assistant in Zürich, influenced Freud, developed the first experimental method using association of words in the exploration of pathological unconscious nucleus or complexes (18). Sullivan said: the mental illness is produced by abnormal interpersonal relations and should be treated correcting those relations but in a proper psycho-social context.

Adolf Meyer considered schizophrenic conduct as a result of a personal history with roots in physical, psychological, and social aberrations and every patient was a different project, the resurgence of moral, humane treatment commenced a little before the Second World War and took impetus during the same war which facilitated the experimentation with new techniques, the Marlborough program initiated in 1938 by Joshua Bierer, was developed then. Its main points were: social club, day and night centres of treatment, mobile clinics and rehabilitation programs. After the war various English medical superintendents directed by Bell, Rees and MacMillan repeated the Pinel experiment in the postwar. They began once more with the moral and humanistic treatment. Simultaneously and under the influence of Maxwell Jones, reference to in a system of treatment and social organization based on the policy of open doors: meetings every day with the active participation of patients in administrative decisions, occupational, recreational and social activities (16). In Amsterdam, this program was implemented with visits to help patients with medicines and therapies of support. This program was very successful: some patients no longer needed hospitalization. The superintendents of hospitals in North America interested in the issue, started organizing conferences, visits to England funded by Milbank Memorial Foundation and repeated the European example.

In 1961, Goffman in his book Asylum, describes a hospital as a citadel isolated from the rest of society. This is a "total institution" as he called it; and it is integrated by two social classes: one dominant and the other dominated. When both interact, a process of dehumanization started, ending with a total loss of the individual identity (10).

The Mental Hospital, another study by Stanto and Schwartz, studied a prestigious private hospital to see its social structure and examined the social interaction among employees, employees and patients, and between patients. A basic conclusion was that for every conflict at personal level there was a loss of functional capability in patients who suffered a severe regression (27). In 1961, The American Society for Public Health, described the Social Breakdown Syndrome, which is a particular form of social incapability as a result of a long confinement in hospitals.

In the USA, Pasamanick and associates demonstrated that many chronic schizophrenics may be assisted without hospitalization, in their own residences with regular visits.

At this stage, the introduction of chlorpromazine revolutionized the traditional methods of treatment. It is important, however, to indicate that community psychiatry was not the result of the chlorpromazine but preceded it. The introduction of the phenothiazines allowed many chronic patients to leave the hospital.

In 1955, the American Congress accepted the Mental Health Study Act, recommending the formation of an Action for Mental Health Act that in 1961, proposed that the treatment for the chronic mental patients was not in the hospital but in the community.

All this went public through John F. Kennedy on February 5, 1963. He also proposed creation of centres for mental health in all communities.

Ten years later, in 1973, Reich wrote in an editorial of the American Journal of Psychiatry: "our actual policy of discharging incapable helpless human beings in hostile communities is immoral and inhuman" (25).

In that year, Greenblat in "Dynamics of Institutional Change", forecast that in California all public mental hospitals would close in 1977. As is known, those hospitals continue functioning just like the other state and federal hospitals.

What has changed dramatically is the number of readmissions, creating the phenomenon of the revolving door. Zwerling in "After Care Systems" recommends more investigation on a mobile long term treatment of the chronic mental patient to develop a new technology. He also recommends that the public hospital becomes the centre of community programs. With use of 100 beds and a population of 100,000 people, maintaining a link with mobile clinics including exchanges of patients' clinical and personal histories; establishing specialized services for infants, teenagers and geriatric patients. The links should be extended to legal and social assistance (33). Mesnikoff indicates that we are closing the circle one more time. It started with the individual, the family, the group, the district, the state, the federal government and here is where the circle starts over again.

Six years after Reich wrote his editorial, Talbot wrote another one in the same magazine: "Treatment for the chronic mental sick: continues being a national disaster" (28). Actually in the large cities in North America we have converted "deinstitutionalization" into "re-institutionalization" using jails, prisons, orphanages and general hospitals. So, we have substituted one type of negligence for another one.

Richard Lamb wrote: "How is it possible that highly trained professionals specialized in the understanding of human conduct and with major responsibilities for the well being of the mentally ill make mistakes not once, but many times?" (18).

Problem Interpretation:

Santayana said that those who forget the past are condemned to repeat it. But in this case why forget it? It seems we have massive economic, political, and social problems of countertransference. Let us separate and examine the different roots.

Patients

The majority of patients come from the lowest socio-economic levels; they have incapability problems, depend on public assistance and they have no awareness of the illness, when they get into crisis they do not come voluntarily, but are brought by relatives, neighbours or police.

When they get asymptomatic, they do not have motivation but inertia and do not have a healthy relationship with their therapy, limiting psychotherapeutic intervention. Chronic patients concentrate on a marginal survival. If pressure is applied, they develop incapability symptoms. The less deteriorated use pseudopsychopathic methods to get hospitalization or economic help.

Wing's studies suggest the chronic sick are vulnerable to ordinary tensions of life. Too much stimulus, may decompensate them and lack of stimulus may bring them isolation (31). Brown, Birley and Wing demonstrated that antipsychotic drugs do not work in patients who come from emotional families whose interaction is characterized by hostile feelings and negative attitudes (2).

Vaughn and Leff noted additionally the tendency to the discord and overprotection (30). Another group of patients show resistance to the psychopharmacologic regimen prescribed because of some psychotic symptoms such as hypomanic excitation. Paul says that only 6% of patients who have been hospitalized, are capable of adaptation which permits them to live out of hospitals. This data has not changed in the last 100 years.

Therapist

The majority of therapists come from the middle class and they bring therapeutic values from that class in discord with the values of the class less fortunate. In general, the training of professionals in mental health is oriented to the treatment of neurotic, introspective and psychologically sophisticated patients. Therapists, besides their economic motivation, have psychological needs of curing their patients. The chronic indigent patient frustrates both needs, because if he does not regress, he develops a chronic and untreatable dependence. The therapist defends himself by ignoring him, avoiding him or being indifferent. As much advanced as is the professional training, so the tendency of ignoring, avoiding or abandoning their patient. In general, the professional, for economic and social reasons, prefers the private sector rather than the public.

Society. In general, society puts the patient's destiny in the government's hands. Not only the politicians but also the government base their decisions on economic and political considerations. For instance, in the USA, to solve the problems of the mentally ill they do not take into consideration the scientific investigation but political-economic decisions. On the other hand, the public continues being influenced by fear and prejudice about mental illness.

What has really happened is a change of names for the problem without solving the problem itself. For example: dungeons became asylums, asylums became sanatoria, sanatoria became hospitals, hospitals became psychiatric centres, psychiatric centres became institutes, etc. But at the end, the new home, always stigmatizes the patient's life.

Hollingshead and Redlich found that schizophrenia is more common in low socio-economical classes. They also found the tendency to treat the patient in the high socio-economical class with psychotherapy, however, the patient from the low socio-economical class receives medication and other biological treatments (15).

In "Closed Ranks", the Cummings studied the prejudices and attitudes, the public has in respect to mental illness in Canada. They found a tendency to ignore, marginalize and close ranks against them (4). A repeat study of the Cummings done 19 years later demonstrates, in Canada, in the same places, the same attitudes are shown (5).

Methods of Treatment

After 5 years of investigation, May et al assessed 5 methods of treatment: Pharmacotherapy; psychotherapy, pharmacotherapy with psychotherapy; electric shocks and milieu therapy. Not one of these was discovered to have more merit or advantage than the others. The accuracy of this study, with questions about the opportunities and merits of different modalities, may have excèssive error (20). It should be said that the investigation was done with inpatients. Therefore, it is necessary to have studies that include ambulatory patients to be able to see the efficiency of these methods.

Complimentary Works of Investigation and Personal Clinic Experience

Investigations of genetic and environmental factors: study of twins, adoption concordance and discordance, recent advances of neurochemistry and pharmacology are omitted for lack of space. The investigations in these fields reveal a state of fragmentation. How to explain the theory of dopamine in the production of the psychosis in relation, for example, to the family structure of the schizophrenic? The practical problems which remain more urgent are: recidivism and rehabilitation.

Recidivism and Rehabilitation

Gomez, demonstrated in New York that it is possible to reduce the problem of the recidivism in patients who are indigent and helpless using small systems of mutual help, discharging the individual who does not have family at all, and as a part of a group of 3-4 patients to compensate for their incapability and deficit with the abilities and resources of the others (11).

Fairweather in Palo Alto, studied a considerable number of chronic patients who had been discharged to live in an abandoned hotel. They were divided in groups, and every group had a common task, complimentary to the needs of the total population and the interrelation through the work demonstrated that independence gives better results than dependence (8).

In the area of rehabilitation, some authors think it should take place in the same shelter. Others, however, suggest that as normal people live and work in different places, the mentally ill should do the same to avoid stigmatism and discrimination. We should not ignore the clinical fact that shows that the transition from hospital to community is not in accordance with the function of the patient in the area of living, work and social life. In this way, a level may be transitory for some, terminal for others (32).

Techniques to modify conduct seems to be more effective than resocialization of the chronic patient, styles of life inactive or empty are the results of a lack of incentives and planning of suitable activities. Without reasons to get up in the morning, and with nothing to do during the day, the process of deterioration and retreat make it irreversible.

Sabin pointed out that to establish the therapeutic alliance between patient and a mental health community clinic, the latter should be acceptable, accessible, and mobile. Occasional home visits are necessary in the treatment of the mentally ill. Unfortunately, home visits are considered as a routine work for the health worker, who receives a regular salary and who is not disposed to "looking after people who do not want to come" (26). The reaction of the professional is even more ominous when they consider visiting the home of the patient reduces their own status somehow. Only the nurse or social assistant do this work without any difficulty.

In conclusion, the rehabilitation and treatment of the chronic ill suffers from incoherence and lack of organization especially in the ambulatory phase, in America more than Europe. A recent study from Harvard University about chronic and ambulatory ill with more than 4 years in the community, suggest that the age of the patient is most consistent in prognosis. If the patient is hospitalized for the first time before his 20th birthday, he is practically condemned to a chronic recidivism (6).

Psychotherapy

Even though psychotherapy has been used in the treatment of the chronic ill, for a long time there was always a doubt about its effectiveness. However, most recent studies are showing its importance (14).

When someone decides to apply psychotherapy to a chronic mentally ill person, all limitations of treatment must be considered from the very beginning. The principal complaint, the expectations of the patient and a careful evaluation of the resources and incapabilities within his present circumstances help the formulation of a plan of treatment with achievable objectives. First, the establishment of contact occurs after, a consistent therapeutic alliance. A great deal depends on the therapist's personality, and his countertransference is very important in the psychotherapy of the chronic mentally ill. Without the presence of intense feelings for the patient's conditions and without an unconditional conviction of the patient's human dignity, there cannot exist a humanist relationship. The chronic mentally ill, especially the schizophrenic one, has a psychological radar which detects hidden hostilities, indifferences or scorn. The schizophrenic may be a victim but not a prophet as Laing and others believe. Schizophrenia is not a normal reaction to an abnormal situation. Schizophrenia is an abnormal reaction to an abnormal situation too.

The schizophrenic as artist, philosopher, revolutionary reacts with intense sensitivity to social injustice, but unlike others, rather than create, develops alienation symptoms. His regression is neither at service of the ego nor of society. Before his eyes, society is presented as a Darwinian jungle, dominated by the strongest, the most despotic or the most powerful. It is only when he is taken seriously that the therapist, as Sancho in the immortal novel of Cervantes, will be able to accompany him in a very difficult journey with plenty of ups and downs, lending him, sometimes, through experiences to help him to differentiate the real from the fantastic, guiding him at some other times to safer ways when he is confused, or getting him up every time he falls attacking windmills of hallucination.

The prognosis will always be good if the patient understands that the therapist is not for his individual alienation neither for society's alienation, but for guiding him by narrow paths between these two alienations. The compensation comes not from the patient, but from the satisfaction of the work done and to have defeated fears and prejudices.

Not always are psychotic symptoms unwanted, sometimes they may serve useful functions: for example, a patient got to the emergency service of a general hospital suffering from auditory hallucinations. Without a proper evaluation, the intern prescribed him a neuroleptic. Three weeks later the patient came back asking the intern to get back his voices, because without listening to them he felt very isolated. Another young woman who was schizophrenic without relatives or friends to whom to talk, spoke with her voices. One day in therapy she confessed: "especially during the evening, during weekends, they are my only company". Psychotherapy that combines techniques of support, of learning and psychodynamic principles and that is used with common sense and flexibility can bring very good results. It is self-defeating to attempt to impose on the patient styles of life that do not belong to him. Not only is it risky to stress him but also can cause him an acute psychosis. Besides, if the therapist is blind to his own prejudices, he submits the patient to the same conditions of negligence and abandonment perpetuating a vicious cycle, that we have already alluded to above.

The group therapy may facilitate the acquisition of resources and abilities: personal, interpersonal and of communication. The processes of interjection and internalization are indispensable so the treatment has durable results. In every group's situation there is a tendency to repression and isolation; that is why it is important to arrange one or two co-therapists or have recovered patients participate. The absence of social barriers permits the patient to explore, to experiment and finally to accept the therapists as models for identification.

We should not forget that the family is important in the formulation and execution of the therapeutic plan. It is necessary to define what role the patient has in the family structure. Is he a victim, a non-existing entity or someone who is stimulating, ignoring or sacrificing himself for the benefit of others.

Phipps and Clausen, in a study of families of chronic patients, have found that the members of these families wish to participate more actively in the treatment of the chronic ill (3, 24).

As the concept of the mother schizo-alienating, so popular in the decade of the fifties, has changed, so the idea that families of patients who are schizophrenic are pathogenic, so that, we should avoid them, is changing. The problem of the chronic mentally ill is not limited only to the young schizophrenic. Richard Green, of the State University of New York, studied 1000 ambulatory patients and found that some patients with the diagnosis of neurosis or abnormal personality, became chronic, not because of the illness but the therapy. A typical example is the following: a neurotic man who is 45 years old got psychoanalytic psychotherapy for 15 years without any improvement. This case suggested to Green, first: the therapist overestimated his curative capability; second: he allowed a chronic dependence to make him happy and productive (12).

Not to make the same mistake, it is necessary to remember a very well known phrase of Frieda Fromm-Reichmann: "I never promised you a rose garden". It would be utopian to think that the promise of life and health is a bed of roses.

References

1. Bleuler E. Dementia Praecox or the Group of Schizophrenias. New York, Universities Press, 1961.

2. Brown G. W., Birley J. L., Wing J. K. Influence of Family Life on the Course of Schizophrenic Disorders: A replication. British J. Psych, 1972, 121, 241-258.

3. Clausen J. Social Etiologies of Schizophrenia. Presented at Schizophrenia: A Comprehensive Update. New York, New York, Nov. 6 and 7, 1976.

4. Cumming E., Cumming J. Closed Ranks: An Experiment in Mental Health Education. Harvard, University Press, 1957.

5. D'arcy C., Brockman J. Changing Public Recognition of Psychiatric Symptoms? Blackfoot Revisited. J. Health Social Behavior, 1976, 17, 302-310.

6. Dickey B. et al: A Follow-up of Deinstitutionalized Chronic Patients Four Years after Discharge. Hospital Community Psych, 1981, 32, 326-329.

7. Engel G. The Biopsychosocial Model. Am. J. Psych. 1980, 137, 535-544.

8. Fairweather G. W., Simon R., Gebhard M. E. et al. Relative Effectiveness of Psychotherapeutic Programs: A Multi Criteria Comparison of Four Programs for Three Different Patient Groups. Psychol. Monographs, 1960, 429, 1-25.

9. Freud S. Psychoanalityc Observations Concerning an Autobiographically Described Case of Paranoia. In: The Basic Writings of Sigmund Freud. New York, Random House, 1938.

10. Goffman E. On the Characteristics of Total Institutions. In: Asylums. New York, Anchor Books, 1961.

11. Gomez E. A. Small Supportive Treatment Units and the Problem of Recidivism in Indigent Chronic Schizophrenics. Psych. Quart., 1978, 50, 211-217.

12. Green R. The Creation of the Chronic Patient. Presented at the One hundred and Thirty Second Annual Meeting of the American Psychiatric Association, Chicago, Illinois, 1979.

13. Greenblatt M. Dinamics of Institutional Change: The Future of the Mental Hospital. Bronx State Hospital, 1973, 1, 89-99.

14. Gunderson J.G. Matching the Personality of Patients and Therapists in the Individual Psychotherapy of Schizophrenics. Presented at the University of Rochester, Psychiatric Meeting, Rochester, New York, 1975.

15. Hollingshead A. B., Redlich F. C. Social Class and Mental Illness: A Community Study, New York, Wiley, 1958.

16. Jones M. Social Psychiatry: In the Community, in Hospitals, and in Prisons. Springfield, Ill., Charles C. Thomas, 1962.

17. Kreaepelin E. Dementia Praecox and Paraphrenia. Edinburgh, Livingston, 1919.

18. Lamb R. Roots of Neglect of the Long-Term Mentally Ill. Psychiatry, 1979, 42, 201-207.

19. Lazare A. Hidden Conceptual Models in Clinical Psychiatry. New England J. Med., 1973, 288, 345-351.

20. May P. R., Tuma A. H., Dixon W. J. Schizophrenia, A. Follow-up Study of The Results of Five Forms of Treatment, Arch. Gen. Psych., 1981, 38, 776-784.

21. Mesnikoff A. M. The State Hospital as a Community Mental Health Center. Paper presented at the American Psychiatric Association, District Branches, New York, Nov. 21, 1969.

22. Pasamanick B., Scarpitti F. P., Dinitz S. Schizophrenics in the Community. New York, Appleton-Century-Crofts, 1967.

23. Paul G. Chronic Mental Patient: Current Status-Future Direction. Psychol. Bull. 1969, 71, 81-94.

24. Phipps L.A. The Impact of Psychiatric Hospitalization on the Spouse of the Identified Patient. Unpublished Master's Thesis, School of Nursing, Rochester, New York, 1976.

25. Reich R. Care of Chronically Mentally Ill: A National Disgrace. Amer J. Psych., 1973, 130, 911-912.

26. Sabin J. E. The Therapeutic Relationship in Neighborhood Psychiatry. Psychiatry, 41: 24-32, 1978.

27. Stanton A. H., Schwartz M. S. The Mental Hospital. New York, Basic Books, 1954.

28. Talbot J. Care of the Chronically Mentally Ill: Still a National Disgrace. Amer. J. Psych. 1979, 136, 688-689.

29. Tolstoy L. War and Peace. Chicago, Britanica Great Books, 1952.

30. Vaughn C. E., Leff J. P. The Influence of Family and Social Factors on the Course of Psychiatric Illness, British J. Psych., 129, 125-137, 1976.

31. Wing J.K. The Management of Schizophrenia in the Community. Presented at Annual Meeting. American College of Psychiatrists, Atlanta, Georgia, 1977.

32. Zusman J. Tertiary Prevention. In: Comprehensive Textbook of Psychiatry, Ed. by Freedman A., Kaplan H. I., Sadock, B. J. Baltimore, Williams and Wilkins, 1975.

33. Swerling I. Aftercare Systems. J. Bronx State Hospital, 1973; 1, 104-123.

Fear and Madness

D. Moreau

> Let me explain! Fear (and even the boldest of men can be afraid) is a frightening thing, an atrocious sensation, like the decomposition of your soul, a dreadful spasm of thought and of the heart, thus remembrance gives only the shudders of anguish. But this has no place when we are brave, nor before an attack, nor before an inevitable death, nor before all known forms of peril; this has a place in certain abnormal circumstances, under certain mysterious influences, in the face of vague risks. The real fear, is something like a reminiscence of former fantastic terrors. A man, who believes in spirits and imagines seeing a specter in the night, must experience fear in all its terrible horror.

Maupassant

THE TERM 'PSYCHOSIS' designates today a group of grave mental pathologies and its use, little by little generalized among specialists, is recent. Its apparent tightness and its purely psychiatric reference translates the tentative modern to circumscribe ancient madness of the closed field of the medic-psychiatric practice and to consider it in a purely scientific angle.

Definitions

Roberts dictionary so defines psychosis:
- medical sense: a mental illness in which the subject cannot recognize the morbid nature, with the difference of neuroses (see insanity, mania, melancholy, paranoia, schizophrenia).
- current sense: obsession, fixed idea, collective psychosis, "we have created in the country... the psychosis of war". (Martin du Gard)

Thus presented, psychosis is not unequivocal, but partly returns to a technical medical usage, and to a large current usage which comes from that which is designated clinically by "psychotic states", for the phenomenon cited in example for vulgar use are essentially of the neurotic nature. Curious semantic statute for this word that, according to its usage, returns to two distinct opposing phenomenon. This appears to reflect, besides the uncertainties of psychiatric knowledge, the problem of the status of madness in our century, concerning as well the knowledge of madness itself and the adopted attitude to confront it.

In a number of these attitudes, fear is considered because it holds in these questions a very present part in individual and collective discourses; it suffices to say that press articles or quotes of the type "the dangerous maniac" or "the dangerous unbalanced" are abundant. Also, were we to research, through history, the references to fear of madness and the means of fighting it, some observations on the situation of this problem for the contemporary period could then be made. In all times, madness has been singularised in the community. It is expressed by the difference in behavior; but, by the contents of its discourse, it poses its contemporaries puzzles which are difficult to solve; also it appeals to its systems of knowledge after finding an answer to these three necessities: understanding, protecting, and caring for.

Evolution Over the Course of the Ages;
The Conception of Fear in Antiquity

In the ancient Greek city, it's to the doctor and the philosopher, often combined in the same person, that we address, for madness is considered as a disturbance resulting of an error in judgment or in reasoning which the philosopher can analyze and which he can bear a remedy. The doctor can challenge and address the philosopher, astonishing anticipation of the actual separation between psychiatric care and psychotherapy. The latter doesn't lack, in general, blame on the "patient", excess of passions and praises the return to a clean life, or a better or proper diet to eliminate an excess of bile, for this is known as the treatment for melancholy, pathology which arouses, at the highest point, the interest of antiquity, be it Greek or Roman, and for which the written references are abundant (1).

Since antiquity, the social status of madness and the practices destined to help cure it are the questions for which the recourse to the prevailing conceptions of man and his relation to the world is posed as a necessity. The Greek society rests everything on an enlightened view and the gesture of care would not be exercised without the recourse to philosophical reflections; this requirement of knowledge extends until the delivery of the possible cause of madness itself, which isn't conceived as phenomenological evidence, but requires a philosophical "verification".

A story pulled from the letters attributed to Hippocrates recounts that the Abderitains one day demanded that Hippocrates take care of Democritus, who suddenly become mad. Hippocrates considered an elaborate treatment and prepared his herbs; he goes to Democritus and has a discussion with him about diverse philosophical subjects; now, in the course of this "preliminary conversation", Hippocrates is little by little convinced of the good health of his patient. Thus he thinks the Abderitains thought he was mad because they didn't understand; the letter ends with this remark, not without humour, "We must take care of the people, but for this we lack a sufficient quantity of hellebore". This story testifies to the weight of speech of the philosopher in the city, but equally of a possible recoil before the collective agony facing madness. Madness appears as a phenomenon reversible by a verbal approach.

Fear is relatively absent in ancient texts on madness and the most pressing problem remains that of suicide thus we look to encourage this subject. The relations between madness and illness are complex and it is probably our modern conception of the phenomenon that is to us an intelligible difficulty; madness is not rejected from the domain of illness since the appearance of Hippocrates text, but this isn't the only reason why.

The descriptions of melancholy expose the theory of the somatic sphere with the dysfunction of black bile, attributed to pernicious accumulation emanating from the spleen, but reversible; under certain therapeutic or evolutionary conditions, this conception is an integral part of the system of the "four humors" (black bile, blood, yellow bile, phlegm). The cyclical states seemed to highly interest ancient practitioners, and they are well-known and described; alternation of depressed and maniac states lent well to the theory that corresponds with seasons and the ages of the life. The fear does not result in the comportment of the mad, but more of the dread of the somatic approach degrading the inside of the body (the idea hadn't yet narrowed down to the brain), interior causes could produce diverse illnesses, furious madness, epilepsy, sadness, cutaneous lesions. Galen proposed to evacuate the surplus of bile by bleeding, thus the very black product would adjust to the equivocal.

It's the Greeks who equally named fear and could differentiate it from dread; thus they recognized two divinities, Deimos of fear, and Phobos of dread, of which they conceived to make them appeals in different manners; fear must be conspired with in times of battle to keep the cohesion of the troops from peril. Thus, at the end of the day, refit the terror among the troops and the shepherds; his "discordant" voice would sow the disorder of the fleet from Xerxes to Salamis and would stop the Gauls at Delphi. The Romans made appeals in the same manner to Pallor and Pavor. This division prefigures the split between fear and anguish that contemporary knowledge speaks of.

The Fear in the Middle Ages

The Middle ages, despite its abiding reference to the ancient world, in its scientific and medical domains apprehends madness much differently. The middle ages and the renaissance are riddled with fear in all its domains. Jean Delumeau in "The fear of the west" (2) studied a period of four centuries of which he says: "The accumulation of aggressions that hit the population of the West, from 1348 to the beginning of the 17th century, created, from the top to the bottom of the social scale, a profound psychic tremor which would testify in all languages of the time, words and pictures. A 'country of fear' was constituted, of inside which a civilization felt unease and which populated with morbid fantasies" (3).

The origin of this great fear stemmed from very real plagues, the pestilence which totally covered this period and that of the great wars: Hundred Years War, then Wars of Religions. In this atmosphere a sort of secondary fear appeared, that of the devil and of possession: "...the 11th and 12th centuries saw produced, at least in the west, the first 'diabolical explosion' (J. LeGoff) who illustrates, for us, Satan with red eyes, with hair and wings of the fire of the Apocalypse of Saint-Sever, the devil man-eater of Saint-Pierre-de-

Chauvigny, the immense demons of Autun, the infernal creatures who, at Vezelay, at Moissac or at Saint-Benoit-sur-Loire, possess and torture humans. Assimilated by the feudal code to a disloyal vassal, Satan thus makes his grand entrance into our civilization"(4).

The fear of Satan permits the understanding of the development of sorcery and the role to which the church is attributed as a reassuring and protective institution. In the number of diabolical manifestations, possession and its diverse physical expressions rapidly pose the investigative problem of distinguishing between those possessed and those falsely possessed, preoccupation with a peripheral purpose, and the excess of the inquisition ends by posing as humanitarian necessities. The procedure thus integrates the study of madness and the recourse to medicine as a current practice. The proximity of madness and of diabolical possession does not linger less, and for a long time, a question not entirely resolved, was whether the devil takes possession of the bodies of victims and produces diverse manifestations, physical or mental, and whether the beings of malevolent undertakings tempt and mislead men from the road of trust, by their unusual discourse.

Artistic and literary productions from the end of the middle ages and the renaissance juxtaposed madness and sorcery; thus Brant, in his "Nave of the mad" of 1494, recounts a maritime voyage of the mad, leaving without a map or compass, in search of the "land of plenty", an illusory paradise that the mad would never reach and thus the search would lead them to death. Jerome Bosch, in the "Temptation of Saint-Antoine", we see a dreamlike vision universe, nearly hallucinating, showing the saint confronting the universe of madness. To give justice to the middle ages, it perhaps functions as a return to a primitive Christian tradition, as it appears in the Apocalypse of Saint-Jean and in the temptations of Christ in the desert.

The devil is the author of these visions; he is the creator of the physical transformations of the Lycanthropes; he induces the alterations of the senses, be it by madness, be it by the creations of gifts and extraordinary capacities. This demonological discourse is the object of "Malleus Maleficarum" (The Witches' Hammer) by H. Institoris (Kraemer) and J. Spenger (5), a true manual of the inquisitors. In this type of work, we restore the concern of differentiating between witches and mad people. Jean Bodin (6), author in 1580 of "The Demonomanie of Witches" advises to mistrust those who confess too easily; he sees in them suicidals who look only to die. Johann Weyer (1515-1588), medical doctor at the University of Paris published an important work "Of the imposture of devils"(7), compiling great clinical riches. He recommends the practice of a true diagnostic psychiatrist in the procedure of witchcraft: "Firstly and above all things incontinent that we perceive badly begot against the order of nature, it must have recourse with ordinance of God, to whom which, being celebrity by doctrine, profession and use, hears well illnesses, their differences, their signs, and their causes: it's the knowledge of medicine that has good conscience." Later on, it evokes the passages on madness and possession: "That we think many are demoniacs, those which are only tormented by melancholy, and on the contrary it became ordinarily that all the demoniacs become melancholious"(8). With this true birth of expertise, of the same movement, madness leaves the strictly popular and religious domain and becomes the object of scientific knowledge.

A little bit later, Montaigne reports, in his "Essays", the visit to a sovereign prince where he observes prisoners accused of sorcery; he writes: "Finally and with conscience, I find them more mad than guilty" and later on "in regard to those who are mad whom we consider guilty and not sick" that: "it's putting your conjunctions at a very high price than to cook a man all lively"(9). Montaigne, in the "Essays" gives us equally a reflection on fear that announces the modern sensibility on the subject: "Presently, it gives wings to heels, presently it nails our feet and clog them, like we read in the emperor Theophilus, in which he loses in a battle against the Agaremiens..."

Fear of Madness in the Classical Age

Our western culture, in associating the fear of madness with the fear of demon, operates on a mechanism of displacement, in the psychoanalytic sense of the word, and this proceeds and repeats, afterwards, in substituting in these different centuries the fears of equally different natures. In the 17th and 18th centuries, the factors in the protection against madness, in part for those individuals of some value, to the letter of the seal, which associates, in its applications, mad and wanton. The putting to work of the same regime, this of the general hospital, for these two subjects associate the discourse of madness and the subversive discourse and stigmatize in the eyes of the people, like they were of the identical nature. This amalgam, that we could put in the ranks of a true technique of disinformation, in conjuring one and the other of the social life, claiming to protect the people of plague, but aims, in effect, to the security of the state and the protection of influential families opposed to subversive ideas. It must speak with regard to the birth of a project of social hygiene that the development of the state of modern right justifies and imposes; the stain of protection against madness would not be left to the forces of the church with the potential danger that represents the popular movements of the march and the pilgrimages of the middle ages where the private practices fall between care and exorcism.

Fear Under the Revolution

In the classic age, managing madness became a question for the state. This process is contemporary with the birth of the modern state and in light of a developing a concept of the world centered on the predominance of reason in all domains, leaves an open field for the royal state on its domain which integrate with difficulty new philosophical concepts. The evolution of the status of madness and its related social behaviors stays coagulated up until the revolution.

Jacques Postel in his "Genese of psychiatry" discloses that which he calls the "Pinelien myth" according to which the illustrious Pinel is presented as a liberator of the lunatics, thus he takes off the chains at Bicetre in the year 2 of the Republic, gestures that, in the term of a meticulous inquiry, discloses being a creation of Scipion Pinel, his son. The hurled myth would not put itself out and would become a classic of the treaties of psychiatry and even the scholastic works on the revolution where the scene is generally illustrated (picture of Muller, then Tony Robert-Flerury, sculpture of Ludovic Durand). The "primitive scene" of psychiatry assures the diffusion of this evidence; the French revolution liberated the mad! The fear of madness was nothing but the vestige of the beliefs of the obscure ancient regime; henceforth, the mad became a citizen like the others; but, in this movement, he becomes also a sick person and, henceforth, it is science that would regulate the lot.

Pinel studied classifications and orders the different madnesses; he is a doctor, but also a revolutionary municipal officer and assiduous of meetings of the Legislative Assembly, then the Convention (he participates in the service order at the time of the execution of Louis 16th). He is a humanist and refuses to participate in the Reign of Terror; he was listed at the hospice at Bicetre where he hid himself; this calling into quetion of the amalgam of the ancient regime between mad and wanton is conducted quite naturally with a therapeutic orientation with its axis on the moral treatment using the minimum of compulsion, a process in which the project of reintegrating the lunatic into common society is asserted. Of these objectives, fear is absent and is thus erased.

Madness and Fear in the 19th Century

The nineteenth century makes madness an object of observation and a scientific exercise; the big medical hypotheses apply without restriction to mental pathology; citing the theory of degeneration and of hereditary syphilis. Of Pinel, who wasn't an organicist, the drift goes towards the conceptions or the idea of the cerebral scope being advanced, but equally where the notion of the "social stigma" takes the body. The fear of madness, put to the side by the reformers of the French Revolution and that the positivism of the 19th century ignores, reappears in a diffused but haunting form, that of the social peril and the fear of contamination; the spirits are stricken with their functions, but the bodies are insidiously infiltrated, like by the treponema. More grave yet, the theories of degeneration amalgamate madness and its hereditary sphere, opening the door to theories of eugenism and of social control. Having a mad person in the family becomes a shame and incites segregation and the banishment of lunatics. The term lunatic, issued in the century, illustrates well the reality of the social marginalization in a world where the notion of efficacy and of security in the management of patrimony becomes essential. The lunatic himself, who portrays his only fate, becomes the bearer of a family responsibility, that of a suspicion carried by the present family and of the one to come. This far too heavy weight might lead the individual to become the agent of his own demise so much that the confrontation with this new compulsion is unbearable for him.

Fear and Anguish: Two Very Close Notions

This historic outline emphasizes a certain universality of collective mechanisms that permit to face this fear of madness that we spoke of and that we can never directly express. Societies in calling for this purpose, to those they judge the most powerful "ideological" references in the course of the given century, medical-philosophy for the Greeks, religion in the middle ages and the renaissance, strong state in the classical age, scientific positivism in the last century.

Fear itself, a sudden historic mutation, passes from a collective register to an individual register; ancient fear permits the appeal to powerful collective manifestations of strife against madness as do pilgrimages and prayers. The community names its fear and makes an appeal, collectively, to the forces of the hereafter where plays the struggle of the forces between good and evil, that we situate in mythology or in the Christian universe.

The scientific revolution, heir of the French Revolution, confines this struggle to the individual domain and separates the ancient notion of fear by creating the concept of anguish. Here we do not restore in cause the relevance of the notion of anguish, but we examine the significance of its arrival in a determined moment. It is the individual psychological science that authorizes this creation in opposing fear, reaction to real objective situations (threat, aggression) and anguish which plays by the relation to imaginary objects; but this separation, of real semeiologic value, finds its limits. In effect, it is the current observation that observes that anguish precedes a real fear and prepares it often. Anguish, which precedes an action of war, doesn't yet have a real object and thus plays with an imaginary anticipation. Fear sometimes happens in space in connection to the action in case (fear after an accident) and the collective phenomena put into play an intricacy of the two mechanisms; panic, which grips a crowd after a criminal attack, happens, say specialists, in a population which didn't always manifest its fear on the blow, but recoups itself after the blow when the real danger has become imaginary. The anguish-fear distinction is thus, for us, of little interest and sheds no light on the question of attitudes resulting in the fear of madness.

If, as Masud Khan affirms, "No one can express his madness", we can say that no one can tell of his fear of madness. Thus, perhaps it explains the observation that madness involves the advantage of the laugh and derision to the admission of fear. Face to face with the truth can't be supported but the price of recourse to its defense mechanisms; before reaching madness is, in effect, of a radically different nature of which, bodily, creates the sickness. It acts as a wound of the narcissistic nature which is intolerable. If we could support the difficult confrontation of a stricken body, the degree of the effect would be to us perceptible, for it would be appreciable on the phenomenological plan. The effect of the cause of madness is the same as being, in its global existence where, for our sense, all signs are destructive of being in its totality. It acts as the cause of unconscious reactions where the projective identification and primitive anguishes are prominent.

Conclusion

Formerly, the group helped the individual to defend himself from fear; they put into place the instruments of the protective rite and called, for this purpose, to the resources of myth. The modern scientific society no longer authorizes actions such as this; they substitute it with instruments of care of great value; but in depriving the individual of these ancient protections, it substitutes, to the collective fear, an intolerable individual anguish. Thus this probably explains the fact of the principal dread inspired by the lunatics of ancient society was that of a delivery in case of the order of the world (diabolical interference in a community of believers); that of modern society is that of violence which we don't find, in history, other than a few testimonies. The fear of madness is substituted with that of fear in its own person and of the ancient meditations followed by an anguished exclusion often generated by reciprocal violence.

Remember that...

Fear of madness is a universal reaction; it is of all times and all cultures. Historic research reveals that the means of facing it have taken different forms; formerly, the group had helped the individual to defend himself from his fear using myth and religion.

With modern scientific developments, the emphasis is put on the technique of care; but fear, returned to the individual domain, is poorly fought; this could flow into an important general anguish of expulsion and violence.

References

1. Starobinski J.: La mélancolie au jardin des racines grecques. Magazine littéraire, n. 244, juillet- aout, 1987.

2. Delumeau J.: La peur en occident. Paris, 1978.
3. Delumeau J.: Idem, p. 39.

4. Delumeau J.: Idem, p. 305.

5. Institoris H. et Springer J.: Malleus maleficarum, 1re ed. 1486 (trad. A. Danet sous le tire "Le marteau des sorcières", Plon , Paris 1968.

6. Bodin J.: La démonomanie des sorciers. Paris 1580.

7. Wier J.: De l'imposture des diables. Analectes Théraplix, hors commerce.

8. Wier J.: Idem.

9. Montaigne. Essais, t. III, pp. 281 à 283, Édition de 1725.

10. Postel J.: Genèse de la psychiatrie, Le sycomore, 1981.

11. Pinel P.: Tableau général des fous à Bicetre in: Semelaigne R., 1794, cite par J. Postel.

12. Masud Khan.: Personne ne peut dire sa folie. Nouvelle revue de Psycanalyse, Gallimard, n. 23.

Acedia or the Depressed Between Sin and Illness

J. Alliez and J-P. Huber

Summary: Acedia is a term of the classical Greek vocabulary that a Christian author of the 4th century, Evagrius the Pontic, uses in a special sense, to describe a mental state characterized among other things, by disgust and dejection, and which, according to him, falls into what became the first list of deadly sins.

The word was conveyed to us by another monk of the Egyptian deserts, John Cassian, with a change of meaning which made it very difficult to distinguish from sadness: his audience being very different from his predecessor's as he wrote for Latins, was little inclined to anchorite life but among which developed the first great cenobite institutions of the West.

One century later, Pope Gregory the Great removed acedia from the list of deadly sins, either because he did not distinguish it from sadness (and laziness) or because he considered it an unhealthy state and, as such, dependent on medical care.

The word has nevertheless survived until Thomas Aquinas and later, and its study provides valuable data on the mental states prefiguring our modern depressions.

1. *Introduction*

THE TERM ACEDIA, applied to the pathology, remains poorly marked out, and even more, a little obsolete.

It was used, here and there, in classic Antiquity and the translation of the Old Testament, later in the first Christian writings, with a psychological acceptance. It was, above all, employed since the 4th century, by the authors seeing the obstacles of the ideal monastic, in the descriptions of the "vitia" constituting the deadly sins, to the pathological limits. Evagrius the Pontic (345-399) and John Cassian (365-432) described with a remarkable precision - as we can say in a manner of the clinical picture - the essential six characteristics separating them, and linked to monastic life is acedia.

But the later commentators were not more precise with the boundaries of this one, in particular with the "sorrowful". It extends beyond the conventual life and finishes by progressively integrating and disappearing in the vast domain which we now call depressive states.

The etymology offers interesting information on the significance of this curious term.

It comes from the verb "Kedo", which in the active sense signifies "hurt", "injured", "troubled". It is more willingly used in the ordinary sense since Homer, "to worry about", "to be anxious", "to take care of". The noun form most important is "Kedos", "care", "worry", which specializes two particular uses, "mourning, honors rendered to one dead", or "union, parented by alliance" (1).

"Akedes" has, according to Homer, the passive sense of "neglected, thus we do not occupy ourselves with it" and notably "to whom we do not render funeral honors." It does not show the Greek "akedeia" or "akedia" features. It is used by Cicero, and also in the Greek version of the Bible known under the name "Septuagint" (notably in "Psalms" 119, 28 and in "Ecclisiastes" 29,5): it is generally translated as chagrin or sadness (2).

We find it equally used in the first Christian writings, always with that sense of discouragement. It is thus that it figures in Hermes' "Pastor", 19-3 (3). St. Athanase Origen employs it in this sense.

This change of the passive sense "that we neglect" to the active sense "which neglects" is already in itself important. However, it is thanks to a monk of the 4th century, Evagrius the Pontic, that acedia would be known by the church, the success would be his own for several centuries.

2. *Evagrius the Pontic*

He is now easily accessible to us thanks to his principal work "Practical Treatise of the Monk" in Stag Edition (1971). The essence of that which follows is extracted from the introduction and the remarkable notes drawn up for this edition by Antoine and Claire Guillaumont.

A. Biography

Evagrius was born in 345 in the province of Pont. After accompanying who he considered his spiritual master, Gregory of Nazianzus, to Constantinople in 380, he installed himself permanently in Egypt in 383. He died in 399, after retiring to the desert, at first at Nicaea, then at "kellia" ("the cells"). In this solitude, monks lead a semi-anchoretic existence: their dwelling is a simple cabin of crude bricks where they work and meditate, they eat only bread, some vegetables, and oil. They congregate only on Sundays, for mass and a common meal.

The largest multitude for them was the uncultivated Egyptian peasants, contaminated by anthropomorphic heresy (3). Among them, Evagrius was "a sort of intellectual", particularly influenced by the great doctor Alexander Origen. He adopted the heretic theories of his, notably his belief in the pre-existence of souls and in the Apocrypha. His writings, like those of other religious originals, were anathematized in 553. Only monastic texts, where hardly we even find suspect doctrines, were conserved in Greek, but often under another name than that of the author. The other works come to us only in Syrian, the language into which they were translated.

B. The Doctrine

Evagrius the Pontic distinguished two stages in the "monk" experience:

The practice, "spiritual method which purifies the passionate part of the soul". It requires five fundamental virtues: faith, fear, abstinence, perseverance and hope, which chain according to a "stoic schema", taken up also by Clement of Alexandria. If it is crowned as success, the monk attains composure (apathy).

For the Gnostic, that's to say the contemplation of creatures created by God, it is the ultimate goal that only certain chosen ones attain.

All of Evagrius' doctrine has a stoic base, but he interprets the light of revelation. The belief in demons permits him to avoid the classic question: how can the reasonable soul be led into evil (5)? The identification of the evil tendencies of demons (Evagrius employs equally well the terms "ideas", "demons", and "vices") permits him to explain the passion, all in conserving the fundamental rational character of the soul.

The demon (or the thought) is not to him the only cause of sin (6): the passage of the act's representation is done by consent ("the sin of monks, is the consent to forbidden pleasures which invokes thought", Practical treatise, chap. 75). The monk that acquires virtues, that is to say reaches apathy, always knows the temptations, but remains unharmed: we find this again in the stoic theory, which explicates in this manner the difference between pain and chagrin: coming from wisdom, they always know the first, but more often the second.

C. Capital Sins

The study of evil thoughts is particularly important for the anchorites: in effect, the monks in the desert, above all the harsh Egyptian conditions, could not be involved with evil by materialism, thus they accedend spontaneously to the tranquillity of the spirit, but are not vulnerable to spiritual temptations.

Evagrius is thus brought to study and systematize the different pitfalls which mark out the route of the lonely. He makes a work of the pioneer: "on this point as on others, Evagrius the Pontic, acting in a scholastic manner, gave a fixed and definitive formulation to a traditional teaching which, before him had a form even more irresolute" (4).

The lists of temptations had already been established, starting with those of Christ in the gospel of St. Luke (Luke 4,1). Origen, in addition, made a commentary (10,7). Evagrius is thus the first to propose a coherent and fixed list, where each of the eight sins is distinguished (greediness, lust, avarice, anger, sadness, acedia, vain glory, and pride) ties more or less rigourously to that which precedes it.

D. Acedia

> Among the 8 vices, that which manifest most and we could say plainly, the originality of Evagrius, and the 6th of the list, acedia, temptation by the excellence of the lonely.(4)

There again, even if it was original, Evagrius had models. As always, in the first place, are the stoics: courage is a fundamental virtue for them and the opposing vice, "cowardice", evident in acedia which deserts the monk to the battle of the soul: "defeated, the monk is a fugitive".(4)

We also find Origen, in the "Homilies on Luke", about the temptations of Jesus. Amid the more terrible, it cites sleep, acedia and cowardice. The junction of acedia and cowardice is of the stoic origin. Sleep is a more surprising sin (8), but it is explained better in a monastic perspective; the monk must always remain awake for the demon can profit by sleep to succumb him.

Finally, in Evagrius' era, astral religion was still alive across Gnose (11). In certain Gnostic visions, for the soul to regenerate, it has to pass across the seven planets and each time has to abandon a vice. Saturn is thus associated with "torpor", corresponding with acedia (in the Renaissance, this planet was still that of "melancholy").

What understanding does Evagrius make of acedia, that he renders it original?

> The demon of acedia, who is also called 'the demon of noon', is heavier than all of them. He attacks the monk around the 4th hour, and takes his soul until the 8th hour. At first, the sun seems to move slowly, or is immobile, and the day seems to last 50 hours. After that, he forces him to have his eyes constantly fixed on the windows, to break out of his cell, to observe the sun to see if it is far from the 9th hour and to look from here, to there, if one of the brothers... furthermore, it inspires to him the dislike of the place where he is, even for his state of life, for manual work, and even more, the idea of charity disappears from his brothers, and there is no one to console him. And if he finds someone who, in these days, having chastened the monk, the demon serves also to increase his dislike. He brings the desire for other places, where he could easily find that which he needs, and a less punishing trade which brings more; he adds that to please God is not an affair of place; everywhere, he says, divinity can be worshipped. He joins this with the memory of those close and his previous existence, he shows him how long life is, he puts before his eyes the weariness of asceticism and like we said, he makes the monk abandon his cell. This demon is not allowed by another: a peaceful state which follows the struggle of the soul. - Practical treatise (chap. 12)

Evagrius' description is remarkable: nothing clearer follows it. We can take up again, in a modern perspective, the principal elements.

The troubles of the real life experience are characteristic. The allusion to the demon of noon does not imply an hour or an age, but refers to "Psalms" 90, 6.

The psychomotor inhibition entailed by acedia is best described by the term: "the heaviest of all". As underlined by the translator: "the adjective is taken in the figurative sense", "painful"; but it connotes also a physical impression, this demon manifests when the warmth "weighs".

The early predominance is equally underlined, the attack is usually made around the 5th hour, that's to say about 11 am. The inhibition involves the dislike for manual work that the monk is incapable of accomplishing, plus instability, of aggression, and finally the rejection of anchores and despair. Finally, recalls Evagrius, if the monk overcomes this phase, the mood changes, and he is invaded with joy.

Acedia ties straight links with the other vices. It is preceded by the two sins of physical temptation, greed and lust, of which avarice is a consequence, marked by the desire to keep more than by acquiring. It is followed by a sentiment of regret, sadness. Often, to that which follows anger (but the inversion between the two sins is quite frequent). The fact of not having can surmount the preceding obstacles involving acedia:

> Do not abandon the thought of anger, in inner fighting that which chastens, nor that of fornication in continually imagining pleasure. On one side, the soul is obscured, and on the other, it is invited to embrace its' passion; in these two cases, your intellect is soiled; and, as in the moment of prayer, you are represented with certain images and do not offer your pure prayer to God, thus you collide with the demon of acedia, which bounds precisely on those dispositions and put the soul into pieces, like a dog does with a young deer. (Practice Treaty, chap.23)

It is most important to consider the opposition between sadness and acedia: the first comes from the regret of those things past; it is thus a normal sentiment. The second comes from the end of a long evolution, of a complete rejection of the monastic condition.

The treatment is thus different in the two cases. In a general manner, Evagrius adapts to the parts of the soul affected. For example, for sadness he proposes a purely intellectual "therapy", that is the representation to the monk that the goods of this world are not real.

For acedia, which attains the soul in its totality, the better means of consolation are tears, the perseverance in the cell of the thought of death: this corresponds well with the speeches loaned to Evagrius in "Apophthegm of the fathers of the desert" (12, p. 57):

> Remind yourself always of death. See that it will be the death of your body, in the spirit of misfortune, take the pain, condemn the vanity of the world, after being able to live the whole time in peace that you proposed, without weakening.

We can say of Evagrius, with the difference of his successors, does he not work as a therapeutic medium.

We must then underline the unquestionable originality of Evagrius, in the list of the 8 capital sins, but above all in the description of acedia that clearly individualizes, principally in regard to sadness. In the pathogenic plan, he is marked by his era, and his belief in evil spirits which often degenerate in Gnosticism. Strongly impregnated by stoicism, its treatment is exclusively "psychotherapy", and sees to finally oppose the "thoughts" of other thoughts (but we must remember that the terms demon and evil thoughts are the same for him).

3. John Cassian

A. Biography

John Cassian was born around 365 A.D., in the confines of the current Romania and Bulgaria, in Scythia. He also was tempted by the Egyptian experience. But, a victim of the repression that depressed the monastic communities of this region, strongly marked by originism, he had to become a refugee in Constantinople, near St. John Chrysostom (14).

The disgrace of the latter brought him to Rome, but around 415, he settled in Marseilles where, under request of the bishops of the region, he drew up two works, the fruits of his oriental monastic experience, which fascinated the western spirits; these were, in 425, the Cenobitic Institutions (14), and in 426, the Conferences (15). Thus he was the initiator of western monasticism, for he had to adapt to the human and geographical conditions of his homelands' adoption of the rigorous rules of the oriental monks. Tinted with pelagianism, his theories were the object of a certain suspicion, still less than their inspirer, Evagrius.

B. The Doctrine

Cassian had conceptions of monastic life very close to those of Evagrius: like him, he separated it into two different stages, the "practice" (for Cassian, it equally must conduct impassivity, but it is less rigorous and precise as to the definition of this term, and prefers to speak in a more hazy manner, the "purity of heart"), and of the Gnostic, on which he stays equally vague.

It is mostly in the application that the principles of Cassian and Evagrius diverge. It is notably reserved to the eremitic regard and worth of life, as indicated by the title Cenobitic Institutions, the life in common. For him, the anchorite is possible only in souls purified of their vices, to those that are capable of reaching the third renunciation (11).

This perfection, as Cassian put into words in express terms, could only be the lot of a small number, and we don't get the impression that his works were destined to those few chosen: even if he believed possible a limited elite could come to not feel again a voluntary disorder of the body, and we feel the optimism of Evagrius, and his faith in the conquest of spiritual knowledge.

C. Capital Sins

Cassian distinguished, as Evagrius did, but without naming them, eight principal vices. The explanation he gave of this figure is complicated and not very convincing: Moise counted seven nations opposed to the people of Israel, that which ended the total desired condition to suppress the greed to which the monk, set back from the world, could never be subject to...

The origin of the vices is more subtlely accosted: in opposition to Evagrius' simple belief in demons, Cassian elaborates a true pathogenesis, in distinguishing those coming from the body and those coming from spiritual causes (12).

He relates each vice to the preceding one, and for each describes several varieties. He recognizes three sorts of greed, lust and avarice. For sadness, he only counts two types:

The first is qualified today as "reactionary": it is followed by an anger that dies, an injury experienced, an annoying desire...

The second, in contrast, "comes from an anxiety or despair without reason." We will come back to the importance of this distinction.

Cassian also distinguished two sorts of acedia, that which precipitates the sleeping of the monk in the prey of anxiety, the other which pushes him to desert and flee his cell.

He interests himself equally in "the descent of vices": of sadness coming from spite, pusillanimous or weak in spirit, sourness, despair; of acedia, idleness, drowsiness, bad-tempered, worries, vagrancy, instability in the spirit of the body, gossip and curiosity.

D. Acedia

Cassian treats acedia in the two works we cited, but principally in "Cenobitic Institutions", where he dedicates an entire chapter to it.

He begins by defining it as a disgust ("taedium") or anxiety ("anxietas") of the heart:

> The neighbour to sadness, this adversary is experienced above all by the lonely, and attacks more often and harder to those who live in the desert. It's usually around the 4th hour that it troubles them, exciting at fixed hours, like a fever that periodically returns, their soul sick from the violent ardors that light it...
>
> When this passion has become the master of the soul of the monk, it puts in him the horror of the place where he lives, disgust for his cell, scorn for his brothers who live with him and those who do not, and he considers them as negligent and not very spiritual.
>
> It renders him soft and without courage for all the work he must do in his cell, preventing him from staying and applying himself to his readings. He often laments on making no progress for the long time he's been there, and he cannot realize any spiritual profits for a long time and is not united with the given community. He thus grieves staying without any spiritual gains, useless in the place he lives, he who, directs others and is useful to them, cannot build or profit from anyone in the way of life of his teachings! Finally, he thinks he cannot assure his salvation if he stays there, and he abandons his cell.
>
> Towards the 5th or 6th hour, he becomes weary and needs food, and he seems to be exhausted by a long road or excessive work, or having passed 2 or 3 days without eating. He also looks at all sides with anxiety and laments that no brothers have come to visit him. He often leaves and reenters his cell, observing the sun is late in going down. His spirit is troubled and gloomy, he becomes idle and incapable of all spiritual activity and he believes he no longer has

reason to leave his cell other than the visit of a brother or the relief of sleep.

> The unhappy soul is pressured by the spirit of acedia like under the blows of a powerful ram he is brought either to give into sleep, or to leave his cell and find in a brother a remedy for his temptations. But the remedy they presently use makes him sick soon afterwards. Because the adversary attacks more often and violently that which he knows makes him turn his back once the struggle has begun, and he must hope for salvation and not victory or struggle, but escape. Taking the monk outside his cell, he little by little forgets the goal of his profession... (Cenobitic Institutions, book X, chaps. 1-3)

This text has a familiar ring, and it is easy to see all that he owes to Evagrius, even if Cassian keeps from citing him. Thus we see certain new traits being drawn, that already show us what the evolution of acedia would be.

In effect, if under the descriptive plan of Cassian brings nothing without relation to Evagrius, no more than in the list of capital sins, in contrast it situates acedia in a quite different fashion In relation to sadness, and we later explain it better than the distinction between the two vices which becomes more and more difficult. Remembering that for Cassian there existed two sorts of sadness, one good and one bad. It informed us on the case of St. Paul (13). But it equally separates comprehensible and unmotivated sadness. In the first case, chagrin can be good, because it comes from the hold of our awareness of our mistakes. In the second case, on the contrary, the despair is noticeable and is thus an insult to all the power of divine grace:

> Sometimes also, without any apparent cause to provoke this fall, the malice of the enemy overwhelms us with an affliction that we could not even receive with our habitual affability the people who are dearest to us and whom we must meet. And the conversation would be normal, we estimate it inopportune and superfluous and respond in a bad way, as the gall of bitterness fills our heart. (Cenobitic Institutions, book 4, chap. 4)

And here Cassian brings up a penetrating psychological analysis, in showing the importance of unconscious feelings.

> This proves with evidence that our passions are not always excited at the mistakes of others, but often by our own: we are often the

> cause of the seeds of the vices, which, once our spirit becomes full with the rain of temptations, they sprout and grow their fruits.
>
> Never has someone, provoked by the vice of another, been compelled to sin if they do not possess in their heart the matter of their mistakes; and they must believe that someone is attracted suddenly when, having seen the beauty of a woman, falls in the abyss of a shameful lust, but more that this is an opportunity to produce an illness which smolders secretly. (Cenobitic Institutions book 4, chaps. 5-6)

Cassian knows what can conduct sadness (14):

> There is also another type of sadness, more detestable, that does not push the victim to turn around his life or correct his vices, but a mortal despair. It prevented Cain from repenting after the death of his brother, and entailed Judas after his betrayal, not to fix his mistake, but to hang by despair. (Cenobitic Institutions book 4, chap 9)

Cassians' view of sadness has a certain number of the characteristics of acedia: irritability and sourness towards others, the paralysis of activity, an "unreasonable" character. Even more, with the difference of Evagrius, Cassian doesn't see the origin only in the regrets of things passed, but profoundly, in the set of the soul. The treatment and the prevention of these two sins, sadness and acedia, are thus neighbours, and we will find them again in Cassian that of the monacal prescriptions: "pray and work". The first injunction is evidently not forgotten by Cassian, who repeats with insistence: prayer is the proof that the monk does not despair divine salvation. But he puts emphasis on the second one more important than Evagrius. He justifies several recoveries, not only by the prevention of sin, but also by citing the Apostle: "may he who works not eat not" (2 Thesselonians, 10) (15).

With multiple recoveries, he stresses the importance of work, which he considers as a religious obligation, a means to prevent the eruption of vices, and a treatment if they are already involved (16).

But Cassian stresses that work alone is not the end, nor is the production of material objects; he cites with admiration the lonely people in Egypt who have few needs, and find the ones they do have to satisfy easily, but still wish to work with their hands: they make things out of willows, and every year regularly burn the fruits of their labors.

The difference between Evagrius and Cassian has two origins:

Cassian is more "practical" in the modern sense of the term while Evagrius is more "theoretic". The first wrote in Latin, language of the law, the second wrote in Greek, language of the philosopher.

Above all, Evagrius practically only looks at anchoretic life, in the desert of Egypt. Cassian, on the other hand, looks almost exclusively at the cenobitic life of the west, in a sociologically very different geographical center.

The "therapeutic" aspect shows: Cassian insists on the difficulties of life in the community and on the importance of classifying prescriptions, notably for dress and work; Evagrius puts more emphasis on individual asceticism and spiritual research.

4. Saint Gregory the Great

The work of this pope of the high Middle Ages marks the end of the change begun by Cassian; the rupture in relation to Greek thought is completed, and a large part of theoretic and analytic wealth that it brought to the Christian religion is lost with it. We will see the repercussions of this change in the notions of capital sin in general and of acedia in particular.

A. Biography

Saint Gregory was born in 540 of a rich Roman family, having already given many religious people, including a pope, to the church. In 572, he was named "Praefectus Urbis", but he retired from civil life after two years and devoted the family fortune to the foundation of a number of monasteries. In 579, Pope Pelagius II sent him as Apocrisiair (that's to say, the only representative of apostolic seat), to Contantinople. He stayed there until 584. In 590 he was elected pope: times were difficult, his responsibilities, more material than spiritual, were always crushing and he always regretted monastic life. Thus he wrote in his dedication- letter "Morals on Job" (17):

> As it often arrives to the waves snatching a ship, even in the most sheltered bay, when the storm abruptly is unleashed, under the pretext of my ordination, I am thrown back in the sea of worldly affairs. To conserve without vigor the peace of the cloister, it is without losing it that I understand how many I have to attach myself to. To engage myself in the service of altar saint, they oppose

> me with obedience of virtue, I accept under color to better serve the church: at this hour, if I could without sinning, I would liberate myself through escape. Later, some resistance that I could make, to this ministry already heavy, we add the burden of pastoral charge. I support it so much as more difficulty now then, it doesn't seem to be the height of my spot, no confidence consoles me, or permits me to breathe. In these troubled times where the world is almost at its end, the miseries multiply, and we that believe to be absorbed by the mysteries of inner life, we get a corner on exterior worries. (Morals on Job, dedicated letter, Chap. 1)

Even more, health was always precarious that which contributed to give him a keen consciousness of the necessary somatic conditions to the good exercise of the spirit:

> When the body is worn out by suffering, the intelligence weakens the night even to the research of the expression. A number of years have already run the course, and I suffer (always) of frequent pains in the bowels: I am oppressed at all times by my stomach; I am oppressed by a fever, slow without doubt, but continual. Maybe the plan of divine providence makes me comment on the history of Job in pain, and makes me understand better the test of the soul of an experienced man. It doesn't remain less evident, for those who see it as just, that physical suffering fights and clogs my application of work; when the state of health gives pain to speaking, the soul cannot express itself as it must. What is the body, if not an instrument of intelligence?

Beyond the reform of mass and the codification of song which bears his name, St. Gregory wrote a number of letters, "Dialogues", "Regulae Pastoralis Liber", and "the Morals of Job". Only one little part of this work is featured in the collection of Christian Sources (18), and, for the most important points, he must refer to volumes 75 to 79 of "Latin Patrologie", Migne (1844).

B. The Doctrine

We are principally interested here in the work in which St. Gregory treated capital sins, "Morals in Job", is compiled of 35 books composed between approximately 579-585. "Homilies delivered in Constantinople before the monks, the true brothers of Gregory, and under their request, the Morals are before all the monastic conferences"(19). In this way they made apparent the work of Cassian, so later, as we see, St. Gregory inspired several repossessions.

As much as the title of the work announces the commentary of a canonical text, the loose manner of the author relates his suggestions on a subject in a true treatise of theology.

The difference with the predecessors, Greek or even Latin, is striking. In his time, troubled and marked with catastrophes of all sorts, St. Gregory inherited the definitive break with ancient culture: despite his long stay in the orthodox capital, he almost totally ignored the Greek. Even more, "in a general manner, he had contempt for the Greeks and was distrustful: he is eminently Roman" (20). In his era, the last scholars like Boece and Cassiodorus, were still maintaining some links with classic authors, be they dead, or very old. Even if it was wrong that St. Gregory was, as they would later accuse him of, deliberately destroying the works of pagan writers, it is certain that he did not know them, nor liked them and he never cites them in his many works: "How," he asked himself, "can the same mouth join the praises of Christ with those of Jupiter?" (Letter to bishop Didier of Vienna) (pg. 154).

We are then, like St. Gregory himself, for we have the same feeling, before an ending world. The Platonic or Stoic influences that we can discern in his works are not more direct: they are integrated in the patrimony of the church. The subsequent weakening of his theoretic reflections brings at least the great debates of the golden age or the patriarchal Christian of the 4th century under the knowledge and nature of God and the Trinity. Its other than the general case, as in the testimony of the disappearance of the great heresies his privileged study to the contrary of this subject, he shows that he is interested in human psychology. The extract below testifies to the finesse of his analysis and the heights that his thought could reach:

> To be silent on the pains of man and the fevers that exhaust, it still remains, even in that which we call the health, an oppressed being of a discomforting sort. Does he stop eating? To not perish, he must feed himself. But soon food makes him tired; thus abstinence from it relieves him and restores his vigor. He must bathe to refresh himself, sponging up so as not to stay in the water too long. He speaks of work so as to not draw out his rest. He tries not to succumb to the fatigue of labor. Weary from the day before, he finally sleeps: drifting into sleep, he rouses himself and sits up to not lose his advantage in this rest. He covers his clothes to avoid the bite of the cruel cold; he retreats under the heat, he researches and

> resumes force like the blowing of a breeze. Thus, finding inconveniences when he searches to flee them, the health, reaching a bad injury, suffers of even that which is a remedy. The fevers disappear and the pains cease, our health is once again in a sickly state of which the need to be cured is never flawed. All the reliefs we search to wear out of existence are like an antidote we put against our discomfort. But the doctors change a poison when, if for a long time we attach ourselves to a certain remedy, we become inconvenienced by that which we had thought would restore us.
>
> On the other hand our soul snatched from serene joy of profound intimacy, is soon gotten down by his spirits, filled with dread (21), deprived by sadness, and soon recomforted with a false gaiety... It wants to know how it governs our body, and cannot do it. We are astonished to see researched insufficient solutions, and it defeats, ignorantly, under that which it reasonably searches...
>
> Seeing everything together, vast, limited, it knows only what it thinks of itself: if it wasn't big, it would never pose these questions, and if it wasn't small, it would resolve at least the questions that it posed. (Morals of Job, book 8, pg. 53-54)

This sentiment of the weakness of man explains the clearness with which St. Gregory considers the possibilities of struggle against sin, and abandons the whole illusion of an eventual absolute victory (22) in this world and also the right necessary measures in all things, as understood in the renunciation and the asceticism.

C. Capital Sins

St. Gregory describes them in "Morals on Job" in books 31 and 87. He is evidently inspired by the work of Cassian, but modifies it under several points. Here are the two lists.

St. Gregory	**Cassian**
superbia	= pride
inanis gloria	= vain glory
ividia	= envy
ira	= anger
tristitia	= sadness
avaritia	= avarice
ventris inguvies	= greed
luxuria	= lust

Other terms: gastimargia = greed; fornicatio = lust; filargyria = avarice; ira = anger; acedia = acedia; cenodoxia = vain glory; superbia = pride.

St. Gregory brings back to seven the eight Capital sins of Cassian, through the medium of an trick under the influence of St. Augustine, he partially counts pride, that he puts as the origin of all sulleness. "But pride, to be a super-vice, is not less than a vice, and the total of eight are thus found, in reality, with St. Gregory" (19).

More importantly, St. Gregory put in the list envy, which becomes a sin for the most part, thus Cassian only has one dependence on pride. This addition becomes possible by the other essential modification, the suppression of acedia, on which we will come back to.

We must equally emphasize:

- The replacement of the Greek technical terms (filargyria, gastrimargia, cenodoxia) with words of the current Latin language, another testimony of the rupture with the past.
- The modifications of order: Cassian wrote exclusively for monks and thus adopts a practical classification: sins are described by the order of battle, starting with the first against which they must struggle and which ends with pride, the last temptation of the recluse who overcomes all preceding obstacles. St. Gregory envisions a larger public, in general Christians, preoccupied with the salvation of the soul, and prefers a genetic order: "The disorder of inferior appetites is caused by a greater antecedent disorder."(19)
- Secondary vices, issues of capital vices, are relatively similar, despite a few detailed modifications, principally consequences of the changes made by the principal list.
- Finally, like Cassian, but with the difference of Evagrius, St. Gregory strictly limits the influence of demons, and at one time, does not identify with passions:

> When Satan desires to tempt a saint, it is still to God that he extends his hand. It is remarkable that he does not attribute to himself the force of striking, he who never misses posting his pride against the author of all things. The devil knows that by himself he is capable of nothing. (Morals on Job, book 2, pg. 16)

This diminution of the direct influence of the evil spirit can only reinforce the carrying of the knowledge of ones-self and thus of psychological analysis, but, on the other hand, by putting emphasis on human weakness and its responsibility as to sin, it takes away all hopes of reaching a definitive "cure" for the soul.

D. Acedia

St. Gregory, as we've seen, made up the list of capital sins so that sadness would be withdrawn.

Two reasons can justify this suppression:

a. The confusion between sadness and laziness. St. Gregory ignores the Greek: The word "acedia" doesn't say anything more for him and we have already stated his tendency to suppress all Hellenic words in his nomenclature.

At the same level as the psychological content of the concept, two fundamental notions are characterized:

- Overwhelmingly, the incapacity to act. St. Gregory knew this sensation, that could happen outside as well as all exterior factors:

> Very often, so much as thoughts seize our spirit that with little pain can bring all that acts in itself in its foresee-ing; thus with nothing realized, it pains under a heart too heavy. And because, inside, it experiences suffering, it is exhausted, even on the exterior, it is in the calm of peace. (Morals on Job, Book 2, 75)

It is even elsewhere that for him a manner of acting frequents the demon:

> Often, the ancient enemy, seeing our willingness to be useful to others in speech, plunges our intelligence into a sort of lazy torpor, so it is incapable to make itself useful to someone else, even when it is free of all personal preoccupation. (Morals on Job, Book 2, 73)

In effect, laziness, above all intellectual, is taken from God and renders man similar to a beast (see "Morals on Job" books 11, 5 and 15,5).

In this context, St. Gregory does not use the word "acedia", but classic terms such as "pigritia", "otium", "torpor" or their derivations. In this sense, he already considers laziness, physical or psychic, as a capital sin, even if he does not explicitly integrate it in his list.

-The unreasonable character, unmotivated or frankly excessive: Cassian had already attributed these particularities to sadness, thus for Evagrius this was simply the regret if not excusable, less comprehensible, of things past. Sadness was thus a long passing of mistakes, inherited from the stoics, that Cassian developed:

> It is sour, impatient, difficult to deal with, full of rancor, of a bitter sterility and painful despair. It paralyses activity of that of which it has possession of and diverts wholesome suffering, because it is unreasonable and destroys not only the efficiency of prayer but also suppresses the spiritual fruits... (Cenobitic Institutions, book 4, Chap. 11)

This explains on the level of derived vices, St. Gregory does not hesitate to attribute some to acedia, like the instability of the spirit ("evagatio mentis"), to sadness.

There is thus no motive to isolate a particular state: laziness and sadness, that which St. Gregory understands, accounts for the phenomena that Evagrius grouped under the name acedia.

b. Assimilation to a Pathological State:

St. Gregory, as we've seen, is perfectly conscious, and he himself painfully earned this knowledge, for the necessity of physical health for the exercise of the spirit. To cite only one example, in "the Morals on Job", book 11, 8, he underlines the role of the brain in the organization of the senses.

Cassian himself, as he speaks of sadness and above all acedia, qualifies them in the chapters entitled "spiritus", but afterwards employs to designate them in the text of words pulled from the medical vocabulary, or evoking the illness, such as "aegritudo" or "morbus" so that, for the other sins, the should serve generally as "vitium".

Another author, St. Jerome, was also subject to bouts of "incredible sadness" ("tristitia incredibilis", "Letters", 127, to Principia), having already put the monks on guard against excessive weakening of the body:

> It is in the humidity of their cell, the disgust for solitude, a lecture prolonged too much, the noise that rings in their ears day and night, will fall into melancholy, and they need the remedies of Hippocrates more than we would advise. ("Letters", 125, of the monk Rusticus).

The use of the word melancholy (written in Greek in this text), reminds us that this affection was at the frontier of the trouble of the spirit and that of the body, and this, since the Corpus Hippocratic:

> When fear or dread or sadness persists for a long time, it is a state of melancholy. (Aphorisms, 6 section, 23)

However, despite the presence in literature and philosophy of "melancholic temperament", melancholy remains marked by medicine. Thus, we must not forget, a temper (where the multiplicity of clinical pictures that the disturbances follow, and do not limit as only sadness): it is thus resolutely of the side of the body. If St. Gregory does not speak of acedia, this might suggest that he assimilates it to a pathological state and so that, like St. Jerome, he can only estimate outside of his own competence. Nothing can affirm this.

St. Gregory thus ends the evolution established by Cassian: he accentuates the morbid character, irrational, that can assume sadness and stigmatize laziness as a sin: acedia thus has no reason for being, so much as the unrecognized of the Greek renders its etymology incomprehensible.

5. Conclusion

We have reviewed the writings of the three "monastic advisors" of lingering Antiquity. Evagrius the Pontic, John Cassian and St. Gregory the Great, provide a rich conception of clinical views, with the opportunity of clinical observations, with the descriptions of psychological states of the soul concerning one of the capital sins, acedia, to a degradation of the rigor of the observation where these "vitium" are finally misunderstood, to disappear in specifications, encompassed in the neighboring states of "tristitia", "pigritia", etc.

But the term will not be lost: it circulates in diverse later writings, up to that which takes the attention of St. Thomas Aquinas. Dante knew the "acidiosi", the Solitaires of Port-Royal ran into acedia. Kierkegaard did not ignore it and M.Cl. Lambotte in his recent "Esthetics of Melancholy" made more than one allusion to it.

The evolution of the concept, in the long history of "depressive states", across which melancholy and its limits thus keep its interest.

References

1. Chantraine (P.): Dictionnaire étymologique de la langue grecque. Klincksieck ed., Paris, 1983.

2. Bailly (A.): Dictionnaire Grec-Français. Hachette ed., Paris, 1950.

3. Hermas: Le Pasteur. Le Cerf éd., Paris, 1968.

4. Evagre le Pontique: Traite Pratique ou Le Moine. Édition critique par A. et C. Guillaumont. 2 Vol. Le Cerf éd., Paris, 1971.

5. Marrou (H.I.): L'Église de l'Antiquité tardive, 303-604. Le Seuil éd., Paris, 1985.

6. Fillion- Lahille (J.): Le "De Ira" de Sénèque et la philosophie stoïcienne des passions. Klincksieck éd., Paris, 1984.

7. Pigeaud (J.): La maladie de l'ame. Étude sur la relation de l'ame et du corps dans la tradition médico-philosophique antique. Les Belles Lettres éd., Paris, 1981.

8. Brehier (E.): Introduction à l'étude du stoïcisme. In "Les Stoïciens". Bibliothèque de la Pléïade, Gallimard éd., Paris, 1962.

9. Brown (P.): Genèse de l'Antiquité tardive. Gallimard éd., Paris, 1983.

10. Origène: Homélies sur Luc. Le Cerf éd., Paris, 1962.

11. Festugière (A.J.): La Révélation d'Hermès Trismégiste. Vol. 1. Les Belles Lettres éd., Paris, 1981.

12. Guy (J.C.): Paroles des anciens. Apophtegmes des Pères du désert. Le Seuil éd., Paris, 1976.

13. Puech (H.C.): En quète de la Gnose. 1/La Gnose et le Temps. Gallimard éd., Paris, 1981.

14. Jean Cassien: Institutions Cénobitiques. Introduction, traduction et notes par J.C. Guy. Le Cerf éd., Paris, 1965.

15. Jean Cassien: Conférences. Introduction, traduction et nates par E. Pichery. 3 Vol. Le Cerf éd., Paris, 1965.

16. Gibbon (E.): Histoire du déclin et de la chute de l'Empire Romain. R. Laffont éd., Paris, 1983.

17. Schouler (B.): L'exaltation du travail dans l'hellénisme tardif. Connaissance Hellénique, 25, 10/85, pp. 33-39.

18. Veyne (P.): Le Pain et le Cirque. Le Seuil éd., Paris, 1976.

19. Grégoire Le Grand: Morales sur Job. Première partie. Introduction et note de R. Gillet. Traduction de A. de Gaudemaris. Le Cerf éd., Paris 1975.

20. Festugière (A.J.): Lieux communs littéraires et thèmes de folk-lore dans l'hagiographie primitive. Wiener Studien., LXXIII, 1960, pp. 123-152. Réédité dans "Études de religion grecque et hellénistique". Vrin éd., Paris, 1972.

21. Gilson (E.): Philosophie du Moyen Age. Vol. 1. Payot éd., Paris, 1976.

22. Lot (F.): La fin du monde antique et le début du Moyen Age. "Évolution de l'Humanité". Réédition de l'edition de 1927. Albin Michel éd., Paris, 1968.

23. Marrou (H.I.): Décadence romaine ou Antiquité tardive? IIIe-IVe siècles. Le Seuil éd., Paris, 1977.

24. Littre (P.E.): Dictionnaire de la Langue Française. Réédition de l'édition de 1877. Encyclopédia Britannica éd., Chicago, 1978.

25. Furetière (A.): Dictionnaire Universel. Réédition de l'édition de 1690. S.R.L. Le Robert éd., Paris, 1978.

26. Ciceron: Tusculanes. Traduction de J. Humbert. 2. Vol. Les Belles Lettres éd., Paris, 1968.

27. Saint Jérome: Lettres. Traduction de J. Labourt. 8 Vol. Les Belles Lettres éd., Paris, 1949.

28. Hippocrate: Ceuvres complètes. Traduction E. Littré. J.B. Baillère éd., Paris, 1839.

29. Starobinski (J.): Histoire du traitement de la mélancolie (des origines à 1900). Acta Psychosomatica, n. 3. Geigy ed., Bale, 1960.

Schizophrenia Isn't What It Used To Be

M. Henne

THIS TITLE, less than a literary effect, is in reality the problem that is actually posed in front of the schizophrenia concept, and maybe also a certain disorder before a reality which still imperceptible.
There is nothing to regret in the absence of the pathognomic clinical signs in the decisive laboratory exam, in front of that which is not an anatomo-clinical entity. That is why, 'a priori', we avoid all etiologic or pathogenic discussion, despite the interest in research in this domain.

That which this touches is partly the rejection of semiologic rigor, those who call schizophrenia almost anything - Henri Ey already said with humor over 25 years ago: " when you don't know what it is, you conclude that it is schizophrenia" - this is the extension which many, particularly outside of France, give to the limits of schizophrenia, to the point of encircling a large part of mental pathology, and like we equally hold to, extend the field of psychiatry to all pathology of human relations and to the psychological difficulties of existence, this ends by becoming most of the world.

In addition, it is amusing to state that in his posthumous work 'the notion of schizophrenia', appearing at the beginning of this year, two months after I'd addressed the title of this communication to Pr. Pichot, Henri Ey, looking to evaluate the number of schizophrenics in the population, counted by those actual committed, increased by a growing number of ill people 'outside these walls', placed it at 1% of the population, when the figures he was given were one out of one thousand (35,000 for 35 million in 1875, and the same in France) so that the calculation, mathematically wrong, is maybe psychologically exact, if we estimate that many of these ill people are not hospitalized, or treated in an ongoing manner, thus in this way providing contrast to those arguing against psychiatric expansion.

But another thing that impresses in a more objective manner, is the transformation resulting from the therapeutic progress in the last 50 years and particularly since the arrival of neuroleptics and depot neuroleptics. As much as we are brought to ask, in addition to the variable effects of treatments, if we must not describe and otherwise reclassify schizophrenics, according to the results obtained, in the same way meningitis, tuberculosis or general paralysis are not the same since we know how to treat them.

However, is it certain that schizophrenia must be modified? Indeed, the streptomycin and the other antibiotics have fundamentally modified the prognosis of meningitis tuberculosis, but not the etiology, nor the diagnosis that is needed before it is to be effective. A stronger reason is that schizophrenia hasn't fundamentally changed, not only in its unknown etiology and its uncertain diagnosis, but in its hazardous prognosis and in its uncertain treatment, disappointing in part because of the great hopes discounted in the last 50 or 25 years. Its thus maybe by paradox that we claimed since the title that schizophrenia is not what it used to be. All that remains is the nostalgia of not always finding in the descriptions of others that which we ourselves have learned and then taught. Its thus more the fashion to see the thing than the thing itself that changed it.

Firstly, what is schizophrenia? For want of being able to answer in an exhausting manner in the actual state of our knowledge, lets go back to what Eugen Bleuler described, and if we must refer to a concept fundamentally different, thus abandoning this calling and forging ourselves another, or many others, if the disorder must be dismantled.

Thus in 1911, Bleuler described "dementia praecox or the group of schizophrenias", stressing that this group of disorders was clearly distinguished from Kraepelin's classification, and added "without doubt this conception is itself temporary." The term schizophrenia, used by convenience in the singular, as much as Bleuler stressed that this group included several illnesses, could be easily adopted, all over the world, in France and elsewhere, for it accounted for this schism with reality, of this division of ego, supplanted the inexact term of dementia praecox as it did not act as an insanity in the global weakening sense and irreversibly impacting the intellectual faculties. It is, however, noted that Kraepelin already said in his 1896 edition that in this dementia praecox, already grouping hebephrenia, catatonia and chronic frenzies, the weakening was more affective than intellectual.

Bleuler's definition was at the time vague, that which permitted the ulterior overflowing out of its original limits, and pessimistic, contrary to the actual wide-spread opinion: thus Kraepelin, in particular in his last edition in 1910, acknowledged the intermittent forms, the remissions and the spontaneous healings, Bleuler called it "a group of psychoses evolving, either in a chronic manner, or forced manner, of a sort that they could not result in restoration 'ad integrum' ". And he added in the prognosis chapter "I have never seen a schizophrenic leave fit to live outside the asylum where I cannot observe any clear signs of the illness".

For Bleuler, the essence of schizophrenia is the dislocation (Spaltung) of diverse psychic functions in the systems of complex independents compromising the unity of the personality thus dominated by one or the other of these complexes or tendencies, accompanied by associative troubles, caused by dams and the trains of thought, resulting in the affective troubles. This dissociation or division or dislocation was the primary negative disturbance which involves secondary upheavals.

The fundamental symptoms interpret the alterations of functions. Thus, the elementary functions:

a) disturbance of associations explaining the strangeness and the incoherence of thought,

b) disturbance of affectivity different from the inaffectivity of Kraepelin with his absolute indifference, but more paradoxical parathymia and discordance, thus we later stress continuance of burdened anguish or in France with Guiraud athyhormia or loss of vital zest;

c) ambivalence that, for Bleuler, is constant even when it is not marked.

Now the complex functions:

a) Autism: this folding in on oneself is an evasion of reality with the predominance of interior life. It corresponds with the loss of syntony of Minkowski. Ey said that schizophrenia is an "illness of reality, that manifests not only schizophrenic who doesn't want reality, but cannot direct his existence to the level of reality" or again "it is not the desire disappointed, but reality lost",

b) aboulia, where the major manifestation is apragmatism,

c) intelligence, conserved in elementary functions - orientation, memory, sensation - but disturbed in the measure where there are associations and affectivity, the schizophrenic "lacks less intelligence than energy".

On the side of these fundamental symptoms, which, for Bleuler, constitute the semiology common to all schizophrenics, and who, limited to this, permitting the diagnosis of simple schizophrenia, there exist accessory symptoms where the associations between them and with fundamental symptoms which constitute the clinical forms - hebephrenia like in Kraepelin, catatonia of Kahlbaum (primitively called in 1863 paraphrenia hebetica) and paranoid psychosis thus the content is not the same for the French as for Kraepelin or Bleuler and their unknown successors - accessory symptoms that are:

1) sensorial disturbances, illusions, hallucinations, twilight states;

2) delirious ideas that have adopted since this era the Freudian interpretations of Bleuler;

3) amnesiac problems corresponding in reality to obstructions and different from the global weakening of the criticism of Kraepelin;

4) the problems of personality when the subject loses his individuality, his identity, his search in the mirror, etc.

5) the disturbances of language spoken or written that we call schizophasic;

6) somatic troubles, for Bleuler, "schizophrenia rests at its base on a profound alteration of the brain or of the whole organism." It is remarkable that this doctrine that we so much as reproached to Clérambault by example is not of Bleuler;

7) catatonic symptoms resuming the classical descriptions always confessed in our day: catalepsy, stupor, stereotype, negativism, automatic or impulsive acts;

8) keen symptoms, that's to say thymic (melancholic, maniacal).

For the French, the semiologic descriptions remain valuable as much as they remain generally faithful through the schizophrenia of Bleuler to the spirit of dementia praecox of Morel, that is to say a serious illness, often amenable or capable of remission but of a poor prognosis, thus the frenzies are irreversible and end in vesanique insanity. Indeed the neuroleptics have modified the evolution in reducing or suppressing the impulses in a general fashion of most of the disorders of behavior and in wearing down the superstructures of madness but in modifying much less easily the hard core of the autistic, apragmatic and athymhormic, so well that the subject appears better, or stabilized, sometimes clinically healed as long as they take their medication, but relapsing if they stop.

Where prudence does not make the destructive prognosis too rapid according to Henri Baruk's warning, and the repugnance is considered as keen schizophrenics or puffed delirious people, that could be in a mode of entering chronic schizophrenia, but that could also be a reaction to the middle-frenzy to of the relation to the sensitives of Kretchmer, who disappears when the cause has disappeared and the time makes his work - where the polymorphous delirious person of Magnan, that I consider a great deal, as a manic equivalent or mixed manic - depressive on a certain ground that we no longer call it degenerate since this word has taken a pejorative sense, but is often stupid or mentally fragile, with a frequent periodic component at free intervals in the sequel. Its to the point that we see a subject who was labeled schizophrenic coming back much later with no apparent signs, we cannot finally think that its an error in diagnosis and not a true healing. It would be totally otherwise if we called schizophrenia a number of limited states, of neuroses, of psychopathic personalities or manic-depressive states more or less atypical, or again, reactional syndromes. We can then find a place in these categories of extensive schizophrenia for frequent spontaneous healings, for rapid and durable results by exclusive psychotherapies, but for us are not really schizophrenias of less than those Bleuler described and thus fixed to himself the always unfavorable prognosis.

One final word on the chronic madness that Bleuler introduced as a whole in its paranoid form. For the French, this remained faithful to their classical concept at the beginning of the century: paranoid delusions of a schizophrenic are poorly systematized, strange, often incompressible and are accompanied by a poor adaptation to reality, as understood, the reality of madness.

On the contrary the frenzy of imagination, fantastic or confabulant, that we call paraphrenia, lives well adapted in reality, and as Ey said the ill person with his head in the clouds but his feet on the ground.

As for the hallucinatory madness, that we've called hallucinatory psychosis since 1911 with Gilbert Ballet, they are well systematized and thus paranoid and not paranoid, and exclude the group of schizophrenics, but it is true that it has forms of transition.

It is the neuroleptic treatment that is the best discriminant and that proves the autonomy of this very French clinical form. The chronic hallucinatory psychosis responds generally very quickly to neuroleptics provided that we pursue them, thus we've shown in 1954 with Jean Sigwald, that the effect is generally less rapid and less complete in paranoid schizophrenia.

Once again we must distinguish these schizophrenias that yield easily to treatment, less than is administered, and those that resist all manners or only modify in a minimal fashion. There is certainly a view to explore, but nothing yet to determine it.

That is why we remain prudent and restrictive.

The Origin and Significance of Eugen Bleuler's Work: "Dementia Praecox or the Group of Schizophrenias"

M. Bleuler

Summary: The source of Eugen Bleuler's motivation to write his book on schizophrenic psychoses and to become a physician and psychiatrist are presented. He became convinced that the physician can help his patient much (particularly his mentally ill patient) by knowing him personally and by being close to him.

EUGEN BLEULER LIVED FROM 1857 to 1939. The book under consideration here is probably the most meaningful medical and scientific work created by him. It reflects his life aim, set in his youth, and apparent in later works. This aim came about under the influence of his family, the position of his culture at the time, and a society which demanded his being.

Eugen Bleuler's Origins

Like all of his ancestors, Eugen Bleuler grew up in Zollikon, which was a small village near the walls of Zürich. Most of the people of the area, as well as his relatives, were farmers, who were also involved with the home-manufacturing of silk. Their income was small, but enough to meet their needs. An unusual "spirit of the age" ruled in their house; up until 1830, Zollikon and the surrounding area had been under the control of an aristocratic government. In the course of the 1800's, the Zürich region had lost many freedoms and rights. The access to higher education and the practice of intellectual careers belonged almost exclusively to citizens of the city (Zürich). Owing to traditions and customs in the life of the village folk, the subordination of the state only slowly lost it's grip. In contrast to this, it is astounding how the country people pursued advances in art and knowledge, and especially in science, with burning interest. The country people found that the intellectuals, ministers, government officials, and especially doctors, sent to them by the city, were increasingly insufficient. (Eugen Bleuler later described the failure of many doctors in his book on "autistic thinking"). The country population was of the conviction that an only son should be left to his studies, to become a better helper and, therefore, better doctor. With this background, Eugen Bleuler came to an early determination to study science and become a doctor, as his family wished him to be, as the first-born son.

Life Goals -The Study of Medicine - Psychiatric Education

Bleuler's image of becoming a doctor would be marked by other experiences of the people of Zollikon: the Zürich University was founded in 1833, and the first psychiatric hospital, the University clinic Burghölzli, was opened in 1870, very near to Zollikon. The first psychiatric university professors and directors of the Burghölzli clinic were scholars, who had international reputations (Griesinger, von Guden, Hitzig). As Zürich still had no academic tradition, people were always called in from the outside. Above all, personal relationships to the mentally ill were lacking. The foreign psychiatrists applied themselves mainly to brain pathology and science rather than individual illnesses; they were also incapable of becoming close to patients because they could not speak with them in their mother tongue. Within the population of Zollikon one ardent wish developed: one of us must become a psychiatrist. By speaking to patients in the Burghölzli in their mother tongue, there was the hope of being able to better help them.

This was well reflected in Bleuler's life; his object was to become a scientifically well-educated doctor and therefore a doctor who could personally care for individual patients. The book under consideration develops this objective: it consists of exact observations with the inner world of the ill. Bleuler's representation, the "observed" is one someone can have a deep relationship with; one who has warm compassion and wants to help with his whole heart.

In 1881, Eugen Bleuler ended his medical studies in Zürich. In the following 3 1/2 years, he was an assistant doctor in psychiatric clinics in Bern and Zürich, in order to finance further studies in Paris, London and Munich. In Paris he studied under the, at the time well-known, psychiatrists Charcot and Magnon, and in Munich, studied brain pathology under Guddin.

Eugen Bleuler's Work in the "Rheinau"

In 1886, at 29, Eugen Bleuler was chosen as the director and doctor of Rheinau's psychiatric clinic. The clinic, named a "care establishment" at the time, was located out of the way from Zürich, on an isolated island in the Rhein. It was composed of a medieval monastery, which had already taken in many ill. In 1867, the monastery was given up, and the building housed the psychiatric care establishment. In his time at Rheinau, Eugen Bleuler gained many of his skills employed in his representation of schizophrenic disorders. Still unmarried at the time, he lived uninterrupted with his patients, worked often with them, and filled his free time with hiking, theater and dancing. He was at the same time the general doctor for his patients, the nurse, and caregiver, and an inhabitant of the neighboring small town. As such, he reserved a regular half-day for surgical operations. He made notes daily on many observations of his patients, and afterwards put their conversations in shorthand. The number of his descriptive notebooks was in the ten thousands. With these he built the fundaments for his later book.

Work on the Book "Dementia Praecox"

In 1898, Eugen Bleuler was chosen as a professor of psychiatry at the university of Zürich, and as director of the university clinic Burghölzli. His call to Zürich only brought him closer to his sick parents in Zollikon. He was no longer simply a doctor for his patients, but also had clinical lectures to give, overtook sociopsychiatric works of his predecessor, Forel (he especially took part in the battle against alcoholism), and he still had many other duties to fulfill. Throughout his whole life, his separation from his patients in Rheinau bothered him. In 1901 he married Hedwig Waser.

Shortly after his move to Burghölzli, Aschaffenburg, in Köln, asked him to write the volume of "Dementia Praecox" in the planned great handbook for psychiatry. Aschaffenburg charged him with the task because in 1902, Bleuler had already expressed his views in a publication on Kraepelin's concept of dementia praecox. Bleuler was happy to be able to put his carefully gathered experiences into a book. He took the task on, in spite of already being overloaded with work, and with the knowledge that he had no bureaucratic help. In order to be able to work on the book, he often went by foot to his father's house in Zollikon with a knapsack full of paper, where he would be able to write in peace for one or two days.

Today, it is sometimes thought that Bleuler wanted to write an interpretation of illness in opposition with that of Kraepelin's. There was nothing said about this; in fact completely the opposite. Bleuler felt himself to be almost a "student" of Kraepelin's work, and in no way refuted it. In any case, he did not block interpretations in schizophrenia theory. (Kraepelin was probably only one year older than Bleuler, but entered an academic career in his early years, and had already written brilliant lectures on psychosis, while Bleuler was isolated for twelve years in Rheinau. This is why Bleuler considered him to be almost a "teacher" at the beginning of this century.) Kraepelin in no way treated Bleuler as an "opponent", and as well as recognizing his work, kept good personal relations with him right up to old age.

Eugen Bleuler already had gotten to know Sigmund Freud in the 1890's, as he defended Freud's conception of aphasia against attacks. After Bleuler's appointment to the Burghölzli clinic, as he wrote his book, his personal and scientific relations with Freud deepened. Bleuler thoroughly discussed Freud's ideas with his doctors, and had repeated personal meetings and exchanged letters for many years with him. Above all, Carl Jung participated in the animated discussions about Freud's theories, in the circle of the Burghölzli doctors. (Jung was Bleuler's assistant medical director from 1905 to 1909 at the Burghölzli, and even earlier, his assistant doctor.)

The Significance of the Book for the Present

After the representation of the background of Bleuler's book and his works I come to the principal question: what does Bleuler's book mean for the present?

Bleuler's representation puts forward that it is important to consider the appearances, the symptoms of a mental illness in individual cases, and after, to make descriptions in reference to particular patients. Generally in teaching books and handbooks of psychiatry, symptoms are not described as detailed observations, but rather as ready-made concepts which the author has constructed from literature and his general experiences. Bleuler was anxious to describe self-observed symptoms of individual patients rather than preconceived ideas of symptoms. He leaves the reader the freedom to reflect himself on the concept of symptoms based on represented observations, instead of giving him a theoretical concept of symptoms as if it were conclusive. With this he often represents neglected, exacting and factual paths of thought and representation. At the same time, he demonstrates how important it is to reflect on not only rigid theoretical concepts of psychiatry, but also to scrutinize all psychiatric concepts during the care of individual patients. Bleuler's representation is further important for today, because it is again and again anxious to find the connection of symptoms with the entire personality of the sick, and often convincingly finds it. Frequently, the pointers to such a connection are small. However, he often substantiates the connections between the symptoms of a sick person, and his inner life. Psychoanalytical treatments of schizophrenics did not take place on a long-term basis at the time of the composition of his book, even after Freud's suggestion for a psychoanalytically oriented search for the connection between the appearance of particular illnesses (for example ideas of delusion or hallucinations) and fears, hopes and conflicts of the sick person, with his inner life. Bleuler discussed this search often and vividly with his doctors and, above all, with Jung. In these discussions, written and personal relations with Freud played a role. In the progress of these discussions the doctors of the clinic also sought after an understanding of their own dreams and traumas. Of greater significance today is Bleuler's ascertainment that a "dementia", a growing devastation of inner life, which usually occurs with senile brain disorders, does not occur with the schizophrenic. As Kraepelin had already done before him, Bleuler stressed that the basic intellectual functions (conception, memory, experience, etc.) remained completely or continually intact.

Bleuler said over and over that the schizophrenic continued to keep a rich inner life, and that connections between memory,, plans, feelings, and methods of behavior of schizophrenics were found in the same ways as in healthy people. The illness of schizophrenia is not preceedingly signaled by the fading or loss of inner life, but by the deficient harmonization of an excessive division of inner processes. This division, with a coexistence of contradictory/ inconsistent conceptions, experiences, and tendencies, will be clear in the thoughts, experiences, and actions of the schizophrenic. For these reasons, Bleuler did not want to include the expression "Dementias" in the denotations of the illness, and for this reason he especially disliked the comparison of "dementia praecox" and "dementia senilis". (Besides Bleuler agreed with Kraepelin that the illness can appear not only "praecox" {premature}, but also in later ages.) Therefore, Bleuler suggested to substitute the denomination of illness "dementia praecox" with the term of "schizophrenic mental disorder", that is to say, mental illnesses which are mainly recognized by the deficient harmonization and the oversized division of inner processes.

The new term differentiates itself in another important relation with the term "dementia praecox": while the last term suggested the idea that it dealt with a fundamentally uniform illness, Bleuler's term leaves open the possibility that fundamentally completely different diseases could have been connected under the former term "dementia praecox". The most meaningful emphasis up to today should be the importance of care and treatment of schizophrenically ill. Bleuler makes it clear again and again that this is a person with an agitated inner life, and that even if he/ she cannot show it, fundamentally feels as we all do. The suggestion to assist the ill radiates out. If one reads Bleuler's book closely enough and knows his works in Rheinau, one also knows what his treatment predominantly consisted of: he was mainly concerned with creating an access to an "active community". What is meant is a long-standing community with constant and naturally experienced confidences in each other, but without exaggerated mutual ties and emotions. The usual activities should concern the possibility of general work and general sociability in free time. The introduction of schizophrenics in an active community forms a very important part of the treatment of schizophrenics in our time. One understands more and more how important it is to create an active community in the clinic. Modern group therapy belongs to this same direction of endeavors. Family counseling searches to make a therapeutic, operative and emotional community.

Today, one is not conscious enough of the fact that the realization of a therapeutic community for schizophrenics would have been formed in early decades and in Bleuler's time at Rheinau much more easily and naturally than today. The reason is simple: in other times, nurses and care-givers in good establishments, - as well as doctors, - often sacrificed their private lives in order to be with their patients. This is connected with the present day concepts of unheard of lengths of working time; care-givers and nurses were widely known to eat with the sick, to be with them uninterrupted (for example, sleeping in the same room together), and above all, to work together with them mainly in agriculture and in the house hold. Bleuler participated in such a community at Rheinau for 12 years. It was only possible because he, like most of his co-workers, was unmarried, and did not count these hours of work. Since that time, this has fundamentally changed, but the basic conception of an active community with schizophrenically ill has remained; it must simply carry the present day reality.

Bleuler mentions almost all other used or discussed therapies of his time, but finds their significance negligible compared to the active community.

In the closing chapter of the book, "therapy", the first sentence begins with the rousing words: "the therapy of schizophrenia is, aside from the treatment of pure psychogenic illnesses, perhaps the most thankful and rewarding task for a doctor...". It is painful, but realistic, that Bleuler has to substantially narrow the meaning of therapy in the sense of his entire book. The most important of these restrictions are: Bleuler had reason to believe that the various appearances of schizophrenic mental disorders touch on a fundamental disorder, which he could only poorly recognize, and held it as unjustifiable to represent therapy as determined when he did not know anything about how and whether, he had grasped the illness by it's roots. He further stressed that spontaneous healing would occur in schizophrenics (or at least substantial improvements) and that one should not self-complacently trace each improvement back to the therapy. Bleuler, in fact (I will come back to this shortly) observed few cures of long duration. But always in defiance; he was fully convinced that treatment possibilities of the time represented help for the ill, he saw how under him lengthy improvements and appeasements came about, and he found the action worthwhile.

The book is important for today based on still another reason: it describes exactly particular appearances of illness, which can hardly be observed today (for example, under catatonic excitement).

It is scientifically important to trace the reasons behind this change in the image of illness.

These essential components of the book are contained mainly in the chapters "basic symptoms", "accessory symptoms", "subcategories", and "theory". They comprise the greater part of the book. Research of the last 80 years has produced explanations of development and results on heredity and individual dispositions, which are not yet outdated.

Another remark on this: the work time of Bleuler during his years at Rheinau and in the following years at Burghölzli was full and completely absorbing. It was impossible for him to follow up on the fates of released patients and their families. Also, in the Rheinau clinic, almost exclusively chronically ill patients and their families were taken in. For this reason, he had to devote himself to a one sided, bleak picture of the prognosis of the schizophrenically ill. This gave him theoretical motives to speak of cures as such: he had reason to suppose that behind schizophrenic symptoms, a basic disorder was hidden, and he had no reason to assume that this basic disorder would be "cured", even if the ill went back to leading a normal life.

Theoretical Views

Bleuler's "theoretical views", as he touched on briefly in his book, are characterized through expressions which are no longer in use today. He differentiates "primary" from "secondary" symptoms, and illustrates this differentiation with the example of osteoporosis. (He had published works on its occurrence in the mentally ill). In osteoporosis, physiological charges, such as the decalcification of bones, assume the role of primary symptoms. Outer effects of the evident illness symptoms, such as the breaking and bending of bones are "secondary" symptoms. In the case of schizophrenia, Bleuler primarily assumes a loosening of association structures in a train of thought to be a primary symptom. With the same reasoning, he depicts the impression of life experiences to be a secondary symptom. Almost all symptoms which are perceived with the eyes belong to this group. Remarkably, this theoretical conception of Bleuler is similar to the present-day view of schizophrenia: A majority of present day scholars of schizophrenic theory suppose that the illness takes as a basis a predisposition, a vulnerability (Zubin, Ciompi, etc.) and a basic disorder (Hubin, etc.) of which the basic symptoms would be described. Above all a loosening of the inner connections of mental life. (In conversations with clinical patients this basic process was often termed as "latent schizophrenia".) Bleuler named brain pathological findings, which were possibly connected with the "basic process". He presumed an organic basis of later schizophrenic diseases. Today such a presumption rests close to manifold brain pathological and brain physiological findings. The present findings of this kind are different and more manifold than those known to Bleuler. It is, however, remarkable that neither from Bleuler's time, nor today, are brain pathological and physiological findings in schizophrenics very specific. They do not occur in all cases of schizophrenia, and above all, also in those of non-schizophrenics. Therefore, today, as in Bleuler's time, it is still questionable what role they play in the disposition for schizophrenic illnesses.

As Bleuler already suggested, and as is supported by most experts in schizophrenia today, that based on vulnerability and the disposition of life experience, the "unity of personality" is put to a severe test, perceived as conflicting and as triggering manifest illnesses. Bleuler already taught this concept - what is recognized today - is that most signs of illness have connections with the inner life of the ill, connections which one can trace and which can bring one close to the inner being of the ill, which encourage our medical efforts for the patients.

Eugen Bleuler's Later Works

In the decades after the end of Bleuler's main scientific work (the above mentioned book) he devoted himself to his tasks as director of the clinic and as professor of psychiatry. He cared for schizophrenics for many more years, and published statements on the understanding of schizophrenia. In his old age, he occupied himself with the great question of biological foundations of human mental life. At the earliest it seemed to him recognizable on observation, that a primitive type of memory and a primitive adaptation to life experiences belonged to each life. He named this physiological basis of our mental life "psychoid".

Psychological Vulnerability - Canstatt 1841

The history of the comprehension of vulnerability, predisposition and psychosis in the first half of the nineteenth century.

C. Scharfetter

> One observes in many individuals, who cannot yet directly be labeled mentally ill, such a high level of psychological excitement, that only a slight provocation is required to really result in alienation. We call this psychological vulnerability, and most mental illnesses attributed to events already have this predisposition. (1, S. 329).

KARL FRIEDRICH CANSTATT, who lived from 1807-1850, in Regensburg, appears to be the originator of the concept of "psychological vulnerability". Feuchtersleben (3, S. 281) then took this concept up. Both authors employ the concept of vulnerability as a synonym for predisposition. Since Esquirol, differentiations have been made between causes due to predisposition (including hereditary causes or a damaged organ), and causes of a physical or psychological type. (2, S. 29/30). This predisposition was somatologically understood as "psychological vulnerability" in Canstatt's sense. The "disposition" consisted of a "poor quality of psychological economy (efficiency)" (6, S. 189) The psychosis itself was comprised of a psycho-physical reference disorder according to Feuchtersleben (3, S. 301). The psychosis was understood as an illness concerning the entire person (7, S. 358); the "I" (ego) of people (7, S. 545). In the search for the "development line" (8, S. 433), led by people in psychosis, the "totality of conditions" must be envisaged (7, S. 174).

Griesinger (4), quoting Olbrich's important deliberations on the theme of predispostion (in view of Heimann), knew the difficult descriptive recording of "provoked weaknesses" (4, S. 44 u. 118), which he recognized as a problem of energy equilibrium (4, S. 44) and interpreted as a disturbance of psychological equilibrium (4, S. 118); as a disproportion of reactions to influence. The appearance of such a trait, however, is so manifold that a unifying descriptive recognition of the degenerating personality is still not possible today. Griesinger was clear (4, S. 101) that predispositons were "distant but large scale influences" (we would say today: studied epidemiologically) were to be differentiated from individual predispositions, in which psychological and somatic constitutions were named (4, S. 117). In the characterization of a person with "provoked weaknesses" Griesinger employed (4, S. 118) psychodynamic thought (defense, fleeing and other reactions). Some psychopathological depictions of conditions were recognized earlier than that of defense. In this way Guislain (5, S. 59) clarified mania (madness) as a disturbance of the mind in order to deaden painful feelings, to fight their causes "whether searching to dim the physical or psychological welfare of the individual". Ideler termed psychosis itself "as the fatiguing work of the consciousness in its reorganization". On this, the "psychological curing process" (8, S. 658-660) and "nature's self-help" (2. S. XII) in therapy are to be considered. In treatment, doctors will try, with modest caution, to give offers of help which fit the individual needs of the ill. The treatment demands an "unending carefulness" (2, S. 105) and should not engage in "bold ways" (8, S. 23) showing a "misuse of therapeutic power" (8, S. 287) on "the individual workings of the psyche" (8, S. 736). For, in that, protective and autoprotective powers have an effect. Such a view does not remain confined to the pure deficit model of a hypostatical disease.

The "history of psychological development" (8, S,19 and 21) of "darkened and torn consciousness" originated as the "legitimate development of the organic figure" (8, S. 27) and is one in a "closed systematic work of art" (3, S. 374). The history of "illnesses" is a history of classification, and present day studies of psychiatric nosology show that "illnesses" are indeed specific to time and people, and are continually subject to change.❧

References

1. Canstatt C (1841) Handbuch der medicinischen Klinik. Erster Band: Die specielle Pathologie und Therapie vom klinischen Standpuncte aus bearbeitet. Enke, Stuttgart

2. Esquirol E (1827) Allgemeine und spezielle Pathologie und Therapie der Seelenstörungen. Bearbeitet von Hille KC und mit Zusätzen von Heinroth ICA. Hartmann, Leipzig

3. Feuchtersleben E von (1845) Lehrbuch der ärztlichen Seelenkunde. Gerold, Wien

4. Griesinger W (1871) Die Pathologie und Therapie der psychischen Krankheiten. 1. Aufl (1845), 2. Aufl (1861), 3. Aufl (1871). Krabbe, Stuttgart

5. Guislain M (1838) Abhandlung über die Phrenopathien. Übersetzt und herausgegeben von Wunderlich. Rieger, Stuttgart Leipzig

6. Heinroth ICA (1818) Lehrbuch der Störungen des Seelenlebens oder der Seelenstörungen und ihre Behandlung. Anhang: Anweisung für angehende Irrenärzte zu richtiger Behandlung ihrer Kranken (1825). Vogel, Leipzig

7. Heinroth ICA (1827) s. Esquirol in deutscher Übertragung von Heinroth

8. Ideler KW (1835 und 1838) Grundriss der Seelenheilkunde, Erster Teil 1835, Zweiter Teil 1838. Enslin, Berlin

9. Ideler KW (1847) Der religiöse Wahnsinn. Schwetschke, Halle

The German School of Schizophrenia Theory and the Emigration of Psychiatrists from Germany Between 1933 and 1938

U. H. Peters

Summary: 1933-1938 German psychiatry suffered great losses, the consequences of which are investigated as far as schizophrenia theory is concerned. Our stress is on American schizophrenia theory, for the bulk of psychiatrists emigrated to the U.S., and after their arrival an unprecedented rise of psychiatry began. Even prior to this time Kraepelin's theory of dementia praecox had, adversely to the English-American tradition, intruded into American psychiatry, seen via the critical eyes of Adolf Meyer. Meyer added a psychodynamic cultural theory, which was followed by an unduly expansion of schizophrenia diagnoses. The phenomenological school was not widespread, and because of its completely different philosophy was hardly understood in the U.S. Its principal publication, "Schizophrenia", edited in 1932 by Wilmans, has not been translated into English. E. von Domarus was capable of unfolding a thorough influence across Arieti, which has been shown in core example. The American psychodynamic school was hardly comparable to its European counterpart, therefore its exponents (eg. F. and O. Kant) were barely known. One of the most important schools of family therapy originated under the personal influence of Adolf Meyer and was supported by Ruth Wilmans-Lidz. Most of its members later joined the psychoanalytic movement. Nearly all of the German speaking psychoanalysts have emigrated. Nevertheless, psychoanalytic emigrants have added little to schizophrenia theory. Their contributions mainly concerned therapy, which necessitates a theory also. The example of Frieda Fromm-Reichmann has been shown more in detail, and a few others have been mentioned. Particular paragraphs are dedicated as to how Leopold Bellak conveyed European schizophrenia literature, others to Frederick Redlich and the stratum theory, as well as Heinz Lehman and psychopharmacology. Starting in 1953 psychopharmacology developed rapidly and generated a "New

Psychiatry", which ended up in DSM III. Its schizophrenia theory dropped the ideas of the preceding decades and, as far as phenomenology is concerned, attached to its further development in Nazi Germany.

Introduction

ALIENATIO mentis, folia, insanity, delusions, or however it is termed, has a long Oriental-European-American history of tradition as well as being a cultural phenomena and literary topic, and a job for the doctor (Pélicier). Only the conceptions of causes and boundaries have changed. However, a constant core conception has remained. It is always considered a disturbance, which is spoken of and handled as insanity, without being comprised of a brain or other body illness, but also without appearing that this behavior is psychologically or motivationally derived. That is not necessarily so. Unfortunately we know nothing about whether, and in which way, the phenomenon of insanity is present in other cultures; among the Incas, or the Japanese before their contact with European culture, for example, and what was thought of it.

Reception of European Schizophrenia Theory in the U.S.A.

The English and American psychiatrists, upon receiving of psychiatric immigrants, were not without knowledge and were much better informed than vice-versa. The first German textbook of medical psychology, by the baron Ernst von Feuchtersleben, appeared in an English translation in 1847 under the title "The Principles of Medical Psychology". The second edition of Griesinger's "Pathology and Therapy of the Mentally Ill" appeared in the English language in 1867 under the title "Mental Pathology and Therapeutics." Both books had considerable influence. The American psychiatrist Pliny Earles (1809-1892) took a trip to Europe and visited a total of 35 European mental institutions, and then wrote about it in his book "Institutions for the Insane in Prussia, Austria and Germany" (1854) which had considerable influence. Earles did not narrow himself to a report of the practical treatment of the insane, but described at length the differentiating care of curable and incurable cases in the then new Prussian system of care institutions. Earles further reported on the clinical-psychiatric instruction, as well as on the separation between "somatic" and "psychologic" in Germany. Eventually, Thomas Laycock, who received a degree from York, promoted a long discussion on the body-soul problem and the unknown, with his book "Mind and Brain: or The Correlations of Consciousness and Organization; with their Applications to Philosophy, Zoology, Physiology, Mental Pathology, and the Practice of Medicine" (1860).

As far as the developments of the concept of dementia-praecox/ schizophrenia, with regards to what was understood by insanity and melancholy, there was a far-reaching historic established European agreement. The psychiatric emigration, however, had an immediate effect after the high point of Heidelberg phenomenology. This was based on the German philosophy of the 19th and 20th century, on Kant, Hegel, and the German idealists as well as on romantic psychiatry. This philosophical system was not current in England and America at the time. The primary field of thought and experimentation of the "phenomenological school" remained to be, however, schizophrenia (Kurt Schneider, 1926). The emigrants, to whom this direction belonged, found therefore a complex, and to them, little comprehensible situation, as was the case with these different domains of science and culture.

At the end of the 19th century (1898), insanity was newly conceived of by Kraepelin as Dementia Praecox in the form of an "image of illness", and was put forth with a new theory of formation. This "medical model" (Siegler and Osmond, 1974) had it's own tradition, which started in France with Bayle (1823 and 1826) and his description of progressive paralysis; and which led from Kahlbaum to Kraepelin. The astounding thing was that the psychiatric world followed Kraepelin, and 80 years after him, no other model of illness was accepted. Kraepelin's model was first superseded through the DSM III (1980) (C.B. Pull, J.D. Guelfi, P. Bayer, M.C. Pull, 1986).

With the reception of Kraepelin's conceptions in the USA, Adolf Meyer played a key role, which is perhaps astonishing considering his opposition to Kraepelin. This role of a mediator played by Meyer has hardly been considered in Germany up till now. In 1896, Meyer undertook a 5-month trip through Europe, on which he also visited psychiatric institutions.

During this trip he was Kraepelin's guest for six weeks in Heidelberg, after which he became very attentive to his textbook. During Meyer's stay in Heidelberg, the fifth edition of Kraepelin's textbook appeared, which Meyer discussed in the American Journal of Insanity with some misgivings. At this time, Meyer had prepared some barely published ideas about people and individuality, whose description of symptoms contrasted to Kraepelin's. In this way, the reception of Kraepelin's work in the USA occurred through the eyes of Meyer's but it was, on the other hand, made possible by him, because almost without exception, American psychiatrists brought up in the English tradition normally did not know the German language, history, or culture.

The reception of the Kraepelinian system and theory was very slow in Germany itself; still after 1898, the concept of dementia praecox was in use. A broader reception was fixed after 1911 when Bleuler's monograph, "Dementia Praecox, or Group of Schizophrenias" appeared, in which he expanded on Kraepelin's concepts. The name "schizophrenia" had something fascinating about it, and also spread quickly in the USA. In the USA there had formerly been more reports on "split personalities" than in Europe, so that there was something immediately convincing when Bleuler termed the illness. Kraepelin, at almost the same time, became as known in the USA as Bleuler, after a translation of his essential works appeared in 1919. Bleuler's reception advanced without knowledge of the original texts. In 1924 the first translation of his textbook of psychiatry came out, translated by A.A. Brill (who worked on Freud). Bleuler's large book on schizophrenia was translated into English almost 40 years after it first came out. This was the situation facing expelled psychiatric emigrants fleeing Hitler.

Arrival of the Psychiatric Emigrants

It would have been very understandable if the emigration out of Nazi-Germany had strengthened already existing currents of ideas, especially with Wilmans' published volumes on schizophrenia (Wilmans, 1932); as this direction had found its conclusive formation immediately before the emigration, and Wilmans himself was among the first pursued. The classical Heidelberg psychopathology did not carry through to America to begin with. There are two main reasons for this.

Eugen Kahn, in 1930, had become Sterling Professor of Psychiatry at Yale University, because a prominent student of Kraepelin was wanted for the position. Kahn had also written several works which had become known in Germany (Kahn, 1921, 1922, 1923 a, b, 1926 a, b). After Kahn arrived in America however, he did little for the expansion of the schizophrenia theory (only Kahn and Cohen, 1932, 1936; Kinross-Wright and Kahn, 1958). In America, Kahn devoted himself much more to a completely incorrect psychology of experience and later to the analysis of experience. Meyer-Gross, who can be seen as the most prominent member of the Heidelberg group (he went to England) occupied himself there for a long time with the Heidelberg concept of schizophrenia. In his late appearing textbook of psychiatry (1954), "Clinical Psychiatry", the classic theory of schizophrenia was given detailed consideration. From this successful textbook description came a strong, if late, impact. Gabriel Steiner, another emigrated member of the Heidelberg group, devoted himself almost exclusively to multiple sclerosis, while in Detroit. The Heidelberg psychopathologist, Alfred Strauss, had no opportunity to enter the English speaking world from his place of emigration, Madrid, and so there was silence from him. Heinz Lehmann, (who was no longer to be counted as part of the group) went to Canada, where he acted as a mediator for published phenomenological schizophrenia theories from the German language. Lehmann particularly worked on his chapter of schizophrenia in the textbook by Freedman, Kaplan and Sadock (Lehmann 1967, 1980), which can be counted among the best clinical reports of schizophrenia.

Elmar von Domarus and His Works

On this position, v. Domarus must also be considered. V. Domarus, who is perhaps still current among most modern-day psychiatrists with regards to his system theories, did not belong to any specific school during his activities in Germany. In 1922-1924 he first worked in the care institution in Berlin, and from 1924-1928 he was an assistant at the university nerve clinic in Freiburg, Leipzig, Bonn and Munich, and in

1928 at the age of 35 he went to Yale University as a Rockefeller Research fellow. From there he never returned to Germany. Later v. Domarus was active in the USA in different psychiatric institutes and sanitariums and finally he led a private practice for "psychoanalysis, psychotherapy and electric shock." In his early years as an assistant, v. Domarus did a series of important works on formal thought disorders, depressives, maniacs, and schizophrenics, and in particular on the abnormal use of logic and symbols. These efforts led to "Prelogical Thought of Schizophrenics" (1923) and the "Origin and Psychology of Language" (1924), and discussions, "On the Relations of Normal to Schizophrenic Thought" (1925), to a "Theory of Schizophrenic Thought"(1927). This theory, which v. Domarus developed under the term "paralogical identification", implied that in the early development period of mankind the logical and symbolic laws of our language were not yet valid, and that the schizophrenic persisted or turned back, according to the Lamarck-Darwinian law, in this development step. His German works, which are very difficult to read, were summarized by him later in the USA under the title "The Specific Laws of Logic in Schizophrenia" (v. Domarus, 1964).

Although the above-named studies always dealt with a formal-psychological analysis of mental disturbance, v. Domarus was given critical commentary from the Heidelbergers, especially Gruhle and Mayer-Gross. They read him, but with care. As an illustration I have chosen v. Domarus's descriptive psychopathological example, because with it the gradual adaptation of German phenomenological psychopathology in American psychiatry (v. Domarus, 1925) can be clarified through quotes made by Heidelberg psychopathologists (Gruhle). I will repeat this example in the form it first appeared in Gruhle (1932):

> A schizophrenic from Bonn asserts that Christ, cigar boxes, and sex are the same thing. An analysis reveals that all three objects are encircled - Christ by a halo, the package of cigars by the box, and the woman by a man's sexual glance. In this respect the example makes sense. The paralogical element of schizophrenic thought also held that all three identical characteristics causes the thinker to equate one thing with another. - v. Domarus explained; Gruhle continued - the affected ill person experienced the same feelings in relation to Christ, cigars and sexuality. (H. Gruhle, 1932)

Gruhle then critically commented:

> Apart from the seemingly obstinately used word 'feeling', this conviction is definitely an experience of common meaning of three objects, and moves out of the sphere of thought disorder nearer to insanity.

The same example appears again much later (1948) in Gruhle this time though, without naming v. Domarus as a source; since immigrated and hence forgotten in Germany. This time Gruhle tells the small story as an example of an unintended schizophrenic joke:

> What strange thought relationships show themselves in the 'jokes' of another schizophrenic: Christ, a cigar, and the female sex are all encircled objects: - Christ with his halo, the cigar by paper and the female sex by a man's sexual glance. (H. Gruhle, 1948).

It is now no longer a "thought disturbance near insanity" but rather "strange (i.e. funny) thought relationships." Gruhle leaves aside v. Domarus's ideas about emotional thought content. Rather he explains how in this example the schizophrenic can be funny; with this explanation he obviously insinuates humorous intentions.

The same example is also used by S. Arieti (1955). Arieti, who was the most recognized authority in the field of schizophrenic at the time, used the quote to comment on the "von Domarus principle" (meaning the above-named paralogical), which Arieti had supported himself strongly in his principle work "Interpretations of Schizophrenia", and which set the central theory of this long-leading book:

> For instance, a patient of von Domarus thought that Jesus, cigar boxes and sex were identical. Study of this delusion disclosed that the common predicate, which led to the identification, was the state of being encircled. According to the patient, the head of Jesus, as of a saint, is encircled by a halo, the package of cigars by the tax band, and the woman by the sex glance of a man. (S. Arieti, 1955).

In Arieti's writing this example is the essential idea in the clarification of his own schizophrenic theory, which he described under the term "the paleological Domarus Principle" as follows:

> Whereas the normal person accepts identity only upon the basis of identical subjects, the paleologician accepts identity based upon identical predicates.(S. Arieti, 1955)

The example quoted over and over is taken from a short work entitled "On the Thoughts of Manics and Depressives" (v. Domarus, 1928). It obviously deals with the indirect, that is to say, non-literal interpretations of the expressions of a schizophrenic, and serves him as a fundamental example in his discussions as to why a "phenomenological way of looking at things" (existing since approx. 1913) had not yet been naturalized in psychiatry; namely "because hospitals wanted to understand directly from Hume falling back on Husserl, under the evasion of Kant." On the contrary, he tried to "initiate Kantian, or categorical considerations into the psychology of the thought process of schizophrenics. The thought errors of the schizophrenic are accordingly of a categorical nature. The example serves especially as an illustration of a schizophrenic's categorical thought disorder, and is mentioned three times in v. Domarus's original. The first of these reads:

> A schizophrenic says by chance we'll meet each other on a mountain slope (that means, in the belly) in order to turn on a canon (that means, to open a woman's sexual organ). We are bandaid to the woman (that means, we cover her), a direct covering, like a yolk is covered by a white inside an egg. In this way peace will come to the woman and the suppleness of her body (she will become young again through intercourse) (E v. Domarus, 1928 b).

After Husserl, v. Domarus further indicates a differentiation between the normal expression of acts of feeling. In order to illustrate what is meant by schizophrenic, v. Domarus comes back to the mentioned example:

> In the first case (of schizophrenic UHP) there is the meaningful act on which an alteration is based, so that if the belly is seen as a mountain slope, the emphasis and meaningful experience is based on the downward slope; if a bandaid is mentioned, the spiritual covering of a woman through a man's sexual glance is also equated, or as the patient expressed, the bandaid is also a halo which encircles the head and he also means the tax band covering a cigar package.

On this, the conclusion is based:

> The schizophrenic thought disorders are of a specific type, in so far as the meaningful act; concerning categorical formation (E v. Domarus, 1928 b).

It must be added that v. Domarus's philosophical language is not easily graspable, and that Gruhle and Arieti are easier to handle. What is meant is the phenomenon transformed by the schizophrenic "taken literally", for which there is no expression. It concerns a characteristic peculiarity, which is occasionally surprising, to see something common in very different things, although such a point in common does not exist in the usual thought patterns of the non-schizophrenic (U.H. Peters, 1978, 1979).

The neologism of the example, however, obviously contributed to a better reception of v. Domarus in the USA. For quite a while (before the double-bind theory) the v. Domarus - Arieti theory of paleological thought of schizophrenics was shared by so many psychiatrists, that v. Domarus, and Arieti, exerted a late but important influence on American and international psychiatry. At the same time, in the USA, the principle of a formal analysis of specific context on the schizophrenic's thought process was introduced, which had not existed earlier in American or English psychiatry. V. Domarus's influence was so strong, that even G. Bateson had to discuss it in the formulation of the Double-Bind theory. V. Domarus, in the first publication on the theory, finally showed that the language of the schizophrenic was rich in metaphors, which he referred to as "unlabeled metaphors", pointing out that the schizophrenic has special difficulties with the categorization of logical classes (Bateson, Jackson, Haley, Weakland, 1956).

Von Domarus had few public appearances in the USA. As a Rockefeller scholar at the Yale University between 1928 and 1932, he used the time to obtain his Ph.D. in philosophy. He seemed to have turned completely away from science. From 1932-1945 he worked in different state hospitals (Rockland, Weston, Norwich) and eventually he was medically active in a sanitarium. Then in 1939, Kasanin invited v. Domarus (forgotten in Germany and unknown in the USA) to a memorable discussion on "Language and Thought in the Schizophrenic"; in which Harry Stack Sullivan, Kurt Goldstein, Norman Cameron, John D. Benjamin, S.J. Beck and Andras Angyal also participated. The meeting proved successful for American psychiatry, as all of these figures had later great influence in the field. At this meeting, v. Domarus gave an abridged form of his theory in English, which was the starting point for Arieti's deliberations. V. Domarus himself, however, did not further pursue his schizophrenia studies in the US.

Psychodynamic Psychopathologists in Germany who did not belong to the field of Psychoanalysis

Not only in the USA, but also in Germany, before 1933 (before the emigration) there were researchers arguing for a psychodynamic approach, who did not belong to the psychoanalytical movement. Max Eyrich (1930) belonged to this group in Bonn, as did W. Scholz in Leipzig in 1930 - he is hardly known today, however his works are still worth reading. Robert Gaupp in Tübingen and Ernst Kretschmer in Marburg respectively founded a psychodynamic (but not yet psychoanalytic) school, where the principle interest was the psychodynamics of schizophrenias and similar psychoses.

The brothers Fritz and Otto Kant could also be counted among the psychodynamic psychopathologists. Fritz Kant, the older of the two, graduated from Tübingen in 1924 with the thesis "A Contribution to the Question of Schizophrenic System Complexes (the case of Ernst Müller)." As Bumke's assistant in Munich in 1929, he described the formation of the experience of insanity, and took a romantic point of view: "Insanity fundamentally means the attempt of reconstruction of an unbearable reality." (F. Kant, 1929). This is similar to the famous allusion in Goethe's Faust 1, also used by Freud, (which for both authors was probably the source): "And the paranoiac builds itself up again, not magnificently, but at least, so that he can live again. He builds himself up through the work of his insanity. What we consider to be the production of an illness is in reality an attempt at healing and reconstruction" (S. Freud, 1911).

Fritz Kant's brother Otto, (who is usually mentioned in the same breath as Fritz) lived in Tübingen in 1931. In his three volumes "Contributions to Paranoia Research" (O. Kant, 1927 b,c, 1930), Otto Kant occupied himself with the special content of the thoughts of the schizophrenic, and he found striking similarities between normal psychopathologically explicable superstitions (his patient had created a person based on these superstitions) and schizophrenic delusions. Kant emphasized the meaning of sexuality for the deluded.

The Heidelberg Psychopathologists made no great differentiation between psychoanalytical and psychodynamic psychiatry. Both directions were held by them as invalid, and unscientific. Gruhle, with the arrogance of the positivists, concerning the quoted textual position, formulated that Otto Kant's perceptions "originated from free poetic absorption" (Gruhle, 1932). On another occasion, Gruhle seized upon O. Kant without naming him directly, and spoke of "uncontrollable processes of the subconscious" which the author unfortunately had mused upon (Gruhle, 1929). As Kant, who had indeed understood the attack, replied. Gruhle went directly to one of his attacks against a supposed psychoanalysis:

> If Otto Kant means, (which no one would doubt), that both an old maid's delusions of love by her masters, and a clinically ill patient's sexual delusions have the analogous motivation of an unrealizable desire for love, then the author is mistaken: this should be immediately doubted for the implication that a causal relationship is at work. Kant is wrong in clarifying my earlier statements, that the insane are undergoing a terrible experience. This would be the error of romantic psychology. There is nothing preordered about insanity. Between the views of a researcher who originally goes back to Freud, and the here (Heidelberg) cited views, there is no mediation. Somewhat later he says - it should come through clearly in all my statements that I cannot reconcile this depth psychology with science. (H. Gruhle, 1932).

Still, Gruhle held it as "remarkable" that schizophrenics demonstrated "a preference for themes, which on one hand provoke the last question and on the other show an unrestricted occupation with sex. (The loss of the ability of repression- O. Kant)" (Gruhle, 1932). The verdict had been made. The Kant brothers remained little known in Germany both because of this and because of their emigration.

Inside the psychoanalytical movement they also remained unknown, because they did not actually belong to it and because psychoanalyists usually pass over or consider false anything psychodynamic which isn't psychoanalytic. However, nor did the Kant brothers connect with the different psychodynamic direction in the US, so that one is left with no understanding of them. This does not change with their schizophrenia research in the USA, nor in the translating of their earliest works into English (O. Kant, 1941,1942). Otto

Kant worked in the research department of the Worcester State Hospital in Worcester, Massachusetts, and he examined cured schizophrenics; a theme which psychiatry has not occupied itself with enough (O. Kant 1940, 1941). Fritz Kant worked in the neuropsychiatric Institute of the Hartford Retreat, on the shock treatment of schizophrenics (F. Kant, 1940; F. Kant, P.L. Philipps and R.M. Stolzheise, 1940); a theme to which much attention was devoted at the time. Very rarely were so many German language quotes found in American journals as with Fritz Kant's work. At this time there was no audience in the USA for a psychodynamic concept of schizophrenia; therefore the Kant brothers eventually stopped pursuing this theme.

Arthur Kronfeld (1886-1941) should only be briefly mentioned in this regard. Kronfeld likewise reckons back to psychodynamic and not psychoanalytic psychiatry. His name was well-known in Germany before his emigration to the USSR. In his text book "Psychotherapy" (1925) he portrayed the psychoanalytic doctrine in a critical form, and in "Perspectives of the Client Searching Salvation" (1930) he devoted a detailed chapter to schizophrenia. This chapter was indeed influenced by psychoanalysis, but throughout was psychodynamically independent. Kronfeld's valuable essays on schizophrenia (Kronfeld 1914, 1922, 1928, 1929) were treasured by the Heidelberg school, above all because of their detailed clinical descriptions of the schizophrenic experience. Although Kronfeld himself saw his work in Moscow as very positive, he could not influence the schizophrenia doctrine of Soviet psychiatry (Sneshnewski, 1977). Kronfeld, in 1941, killed himself along with his wife with the approach of the German troops. Although rumors circulated for some time concerning his death, it appears to have been confirmed in the essays of many of his contemporaries. In this way Kronfeld, although not directly, was also one of Hitler's victims. Kronfeld's destiny has again become the object of investigation in recent years (I.W Kittel, 1986). Others occupied themselves with Erich Sternberg (1903-1908), who was part of the Moscow school, but whom we will not go into here (see V.H. Peters, 1981).

A Culture Model of Schizophrenia - Psychiatric Emigration in the Surroundings of Adolf Meyer in Baltimore

There was a further reason why the German psychopathology of schizophrenia was not taken up. The entire schizophrenia theories of Kraepelin and Bleuler along with the critic Adolf Meyer were occupied with a simple, formal scientific way of looking at things. Vis a vis a scientific (i.e.. natural science) concept of schizophrenia, the social interconnections of the ill were accented by the actual experiences of the outbreak of the psychosis and the individuality of his personality. Models of illness and culture (regarding schizophrenia) were opposed to each other. Diagnoses and resulting theories of signs, and resulting symptomology only had a negligible meaning. This lead to a wider and wider, and more and more extensive application of the schizophrenia diagnosis which again brought about a critique, and sometimes even a disregard for, American psychiatry in Europe. The frequency phenomenon, for example, was clear to the schizophrenia diagnosis of the New York Psychiatric Institute, where the quantity of schizophrenia diagnoses climbed from 20-80% between the 30's and 1952. (Kurianski, Deming and Gurland, 1974). If one estimates modern experiences with the actual occurrence of schizophrenia in patients at psychiatric institutes at roughly 20% it results that 60% of all hospital patients in important scientific institutions were falsely classified as schizophrenics. In the eyes of the Europeans, which the American background was not familiar with, this could only represent a gross misuse of the schizophrenia diagnosis and had to result in adamant protest. This protest had the much later result of the development of the present theory of schizophrenia.

Neither the phenomonologists coming out of Germany nor the psychodynamicists found anything in the USA which they could connect with. There was no existing phenomenological school. The psychoanalysts worked in their practices, and not in clinics, and only treated exceptional schizophrenics. Most schizophrenics at the time were placed in large mental institutions. At this time, shock treatment had not yet been introduced. The German psychiatrists already knew the theories of Adolf Meyer, which American psychodynamic directions could scarcely relate to and barely begin with. Some, nevertheless, belonged to Meyer's circle, which shortly before World War II to the present day, had a strong influence on American psychiatry.

When Ruth Wilmans arrived in Baltimore in 1936, she found several conversation partners at the Johns Hopkins Hospital, (outside of Adolf Meyer), with whom she could speak German or French. Norman Cameron belonged to this group, who would later conduct his well-known research on thought disorders of schizophrenics (Cameron 1938, 1939, 1944). Another conversation partner was Solomon Katzenelbogen, who came from the Polish speaking port of Russia, studied in Genf, and had spent eight years with Adolf Meyer. Despite his German-sounding name he did not have good command of the language, but could speak French with Ruth Wilmans. Likewise Wilmans could later speak with Henry Fox and Theodore Lidz, because these two students studied for some time in Europe.

Besides Cameron, all conversation partners including Wilmans, later had either a narrow relationship to psychoanalysis or turned completely to it, although at the beginning of the second World War attention was turned to the new insulin shock treatment of schizophrenia at Baltimore's Henry-Phipps clinic. There were Sunday afternoon meetings, however, in Adolf Meyer's garden in Baltimore's residential area (O. Diethelm, 1959). Many participants were later reported including von Lidz (1966, 1968, 1973), Campbell (1937), and Ebaugh (1937). The personal influence of Adolf Meyer as a teacher was obviously considerably stronger than the theories of his written work, which were not in an understandable or easily accessible form. The influence of Meyer's theories was so strong eventually, however, that the DSM II had trouble replacing the almost non-existent Meyer's textbook as a general connection for the USA.

Schizophrenic Family Dynamics and Family Therapy

The discussions in A. Meyer's personal environment gave rise to one of three new work groups, which however, at almost the same time, researched the structure and dynamics of schizophrenic's families as almost entirely unrelated.

Schizophrenics' families began to move into the psychiatrist's field of view for the first time. This was not valued by Kraepelin, nor by Bleuler, or the Heidelberg school, and their problematic views were evidently not recognized.

Today not only schizophrenia but also family therapy is a large domain of work and cannot be closely examined in this paper (for an overview see Sager and Kaplan, 1973; Gurman and Kniskern, 1981; Simon 1985). The interest of the psychiatric emigrants in its development is also negligible, so that only the beginnings of the roots of the three developments will be referred to here.

1) A first group formed in New Haven under the guidance of Theodore Lidz. In this group, theories of structures arose out of the psychotherapeutic observation of families. Research of the Lidz-group was shared with Ruth Wilmans-Lidz from 1949 on (she was married to Theodore Lidz in 1939). A. Cornelison, Steven Fleck, D. Terry and a few others were also members of this group. Valuable research pointed out that the family of schizophrenics constantly showed deep-reaching emotional disturbances and that certain structures developed internally in these families. The logical consequence of family therapy stemmed from this, which applied exactly to this family dynamic, because handling each member of the family as an individual appeared to be purposeless. (Some original works are also found in the reader Bateson and colleagues in "Schizophrenia and the Family").

2) Completely unattached from the above group, the "Palo-Alto Group" was working on similar themes. This group was founded in 1959 based on the Double-Bind theory of interaction in the families of schizophrenics. Methods of research were provided to statistically investigate the schizophrenic family structure; in the meantime family research became the main current of American psychiatry. In this way in 1960 the Mental Research Institute (MRI) existed on the inside of the Palo Alto Medical Research Foundation. Don Jackson, Virginia M. Satir, Jules Riskin, Frank Rosman, and the Austrian psychologist Paul Watzlawick belonged to this group. (He first left Europe in 1957). A narrow connection existed with Frieda Fromm-Reichmann. Shortly before the end of her life, Frieda Fromm-Reichmann was part of the Institute for Advanced Study in Behavioral Sciences in Palo Alto in California

(1955/56), and there worked shortly with Bateson (Bateson, 1958 and U. H. Peters, 1987). A summary of the ideas of this group is best found in Bateson (1972). The Palo-Alto group, however, had little contact with the European groups.

3) Since 1957 a third group formed at the National Institute of Mental Health in Bethesda under the leadership of Lyman Caroll Wynne, with a section devoted to family investigation, which was unconnected to research and began to publish after 1959. The connection between the behavior of parents and of children was systematically investigated by this group. The psychiatric emigrants did not participate in this group.

The family-therapeutic concept of schizophrenia remained so long a center of discussion that it came to be known as "typically American" rather than "European". An "American" formation came about with schizophrenia as a pragmatic mental reaction (although in reality this came from Adolf Meyer's European concept) and a "European" concept was considered with schizophrenia as a non-influential brain illness of unknown causes (in reality, Kraepelin's concept, which was consistent with the English-American tradition).

Overall with the psychiatric emigrants, the impression prevailed that there was no interest in their host country for the intensive psychology or psychodynamic of schizophrenia they had researched, and that one must entirely learn anew. In certain ways this applied to Frieda Fromm-Reichmann, although her influence became especially large. She always expressed broken impressions in her personal conversations which were therefore to be differentiated from closer investigations. It is, however now a historical perspective, and a timely, spiritual survey appears possible through existing conditions.

Psychoanalysis of Schizophrenia

After the historical development of psychoanalysis, an early psychoanalytical origin-theory of schizophrenia was suggested. The first exchange of correspondence between Freud and Jung, and especially the preparation time for C.G. Jung's first monograph "On the Psychology of Dementia Praecox" saw this theme as a meaningful (temporarily the most important) position of discussion in correspondence between Zurich and

Vienna. If this did not come to such a theory, this did not only apply to Freud's frequently quoted false assessment of the transferal ability of schizophrenics. There are important reasons for this. Although Freud formulated surprising thoughts on schizophrenia in the "The Case of Schreber" (S. Freud, 1911), and there are scattered remarks on schizophrenia among his works, he had no systematic summary on schizophrenia among his work. For the early psychoanalysts, Freud's work however was usually their only source of information, meaning that there was no important opposition of discussion. Jung himself could not commit himself to a pure psychoanalytic theory of dementia praecox, but rather wrote in 1907: "The Freudian mechanism does not reach far enough towards explaining why a Dementia praecox exists instead of a hysteria." In the quoted book, which is still considered an important milestone of psychoanalytic schizophrenia theory, Jung took up a biological theory of origin:

> .. the effect of dementia praecox gives the occasion for the incidence of a substance anomaly (toxin), which damages the brain in more or less irreparable ways, so that in consequence the highest psychic functions become defective (C.G. Jung, 1907)

Paul Federn worked on a psychoanalytic schizophrenia theory against this, in which the meaning of the mother, particularly for later schizophrenics, was elevated (Federn and Meng, 1949). His cogently interesting theories and case descriptions on the therapy of schizophrenics (Federn 1929, 1941, 1947) generated little interest among the psychoanalysts of his time. (Federn died in New York in 1950). Federn founded his theories on a biological assumption, which is recounted in the following way for the organization of the image of illness:

1. Malignancy of processes (not attainable through psychoanalytic therapy to Federn) 2. The quality of the personality which fights against the sick part of the ego. 3. All additional conflicts such as damage caused by an external factor, augment the strain on the normal part of the psyche.

This theory of split personality, in which the healthy half is continuously struggling with the sick half, has romantic origins, and is held as correct by most anthropological psychiatrists of today, (although nothing is actually split). Federn had an early influence on American psychiatry, because he had already stayed in the USA in 1914, and had held lectures, as well as analyzing influential scientists such as Smith Ely Jelliffe (the president of the Neurological Society of the time) and Clarence Oberndorf (the first historian of American psychoanalysis) (Oberndorf, 1953).

A reason for the lack of an earlier psychoanalytic theory of schizophrenia, which is not to be underestimated, has to do with the fact that psychoanalysts simply had little experience with schizophrenics. Their groups of patients were often of a different nature. The first high point of psychoanalysis before the first World War coincided with the peak of institutionalization of the mentally ill. In fact, schizophrenia was already seen as a sufficient reason for admittance, so that their participation in stress groups under going psychotherapeutic treatment was negligible. In the psychiatric institutions there were barely any psychoanalysts.

When Frieda Fromm-Reichmann arrived in the USA in 1935 after some time in Palestine, she had no experience in the treatment of schizophrenics (U.H. Peters, 1987). Two circumstances then came to pass: Frieda Fromm-Reichmann found a good position at the Chestnut Lodge in Rockville two months after her arrival in the US, which at the time was a small, private institution with 30 beds. Outside of the head, Dexter Bullard, there were only two other psychiatrists. This private institution had the first intensive interest in the psychotherapy of the schizophrenic as well as in the first shock treatments. Prevailing therapeutic nihilism could not be performed in city institutions.

At the Chestnut Lodge, Fromm-Reichmann collaborated with Harry Stack Sullivan, who led and directed, in 1929/ 1930, a later-to-be legendary 6 bed station for young schizophrenics in other private institutes (the Sheppard and Enoch Pratt Hospital, very near to Rockville). Sullivan thought in a very American style; although he relied heavily on Freud in his writing. For the most part, he felt he belonged to the mental hygiene movement, and above all he was obliged to William Allanson White, who one can in no way classify among the psychoanalysts. As a psychiatrist, Sullivan was also self-educated (Perry, 1982).

It is often said that Frieda Fromm-Reichmann owed her special impact to the fact that she joined with the American direction of psychotherapy through Sullivan. However, the connecting link between Sullivan and Fromm-Reichmann was Dexter Bullard, who was friends with both of them. Sullivan, who lived in Bethesda (Maryland), near Rockville, came regularly to the Chestnut Lodge for two years, in order to give valuable lectures on his ideas. These were recorded, and after his death represented a substantial amount of his work, because his writing was very difficult to understand, and he had little public life. Frieda Fromm-Reichmann approached schizophrenics with a great deal of human warmth, and placed herself on the floor with them as if they would not come to her on the couch. She sometimes went through long periods of silence with them just to build contact with them. Such a behavior spoke of the tradition of "moral treatment". Yet Sullivan's behavior in the Sheppard's Hospital was also not yet to be named psychoanalytic. Frieda Fromm-Reichmann later clarified schizophrenic behavior with the help of psychoanalytic theories. She pointed out, in 1939, that the schizophrenic expressed themself with mistrust, to the early frustration of the therapist. But "the schizophrenic longs for human contact and human understanding, however, he fears further frustration. It can take weeks or even months for the patient to become familiar enough with the therapist, that the therapist is accepted"(Fromm-Reichmann, 1939). The technique of "intensive psychotherapy" termed by Fromm-Reichmann (1950, 1959) was correctly described by Hanna Green in her book "I Never Promised You a Rosegarden" exactly as she portrayed Frieda Fromm-Reichmann and the behavior at Chestnut Lodge (she is called Dr. Fried in the book). The novelistic description of this former patient of Chestnut Lodge very much contributed to the legend like transfiguration of the therapist, especially after a successful film was made of the same name.

Frieda Fromm-Reichmann herself divided the history of psychoanalytically oriented treatment of schizophrenics into three decades. In the first decade there was no understanding of dynamic connections, however an excessive interpretation was reached. In the second, the establishing of contact stood at a middle point, and in the third the correct relationships to the ill began.

After that, the psychoanalysis/psychotherapy of schizophrenia developed with much discussion in dominating fields (a detailed overview is found in Krull, 1987). The psychoanalytic emigrants only minimally participated in this. Kurt Eissler (1943, 1951, 1953 a, b) should be mentioned, who was theoretically based on the necessity of modification of techniques, as the function of the passive role of the psychoanalysts as a mirror remained a problem. Besides him, only F. Alexander (1931), H. Bruch (1980), H. Hartmann (1953) and E. Jacobson (1954) should be mentioned as emigrated psychoanalysts who occupied themselves with psychoanalysis of schizophrenics, compared with psychoanalysis in general, The influence of the emigrants on a psychoanalytic theory of schizophrenia is surprisingly small. General overviews are found in L. Bryce Boyer's book "The Psychoanalytic Treatment of Schizophrenics", P. Matussek (1976), and Stierlin Wynne and Wirsching (1985).

Social Strata Theory

After the second World War, it was long discussed whether schizophrenia was more likely among certain social stratas. Faris and Dunham conducted a study in 1939 in Chicago which suggested this to be the case. It was suggested in the 1800's that insanity was a privilege of the idle upper class, but the picture was widened to allow that the poor classes were more frequently taken ill with schizophrenia. The resulting empirical research required great cost to answer the question. A large section of the population had to be examined by trained psychiatrists. The results became questionable themselves, because the borders between social classes, as with schizophrenia, are not easily drawn. The question presented a double challenge. On one hand, at the time, empirical social investigation appeared not to be fundamentally impossible as the solution to a task. On the other hand, each answer could be used politically. Above all, it was anticipated, that a study which demonstrated (or appeared to demonstrate) the discrimination of lower classes would be taken up with large consent as containing available conceptions.

The work of B. Hollingshead and F.C. Redlich (1959) "Social Stratas and Illness" is valid to the present day as a classical certain region of New Haven (Connecticut) in which they dealt with all mentally ill in mental hospitals and medical practices. Here they found that schizophrenia was nine times as likely to occur in lower classes than in upper classes. However, neuroses were more often found among the upper classes. The explanation was very banal; members of the lower classes were sooner confined to a state mental hospital and were kept there longer. The frequently presented theory of migration was seen as invalid by Hollingshead and Redlich. According to this theory, schizophrenics descended in social standing. Hollingshead and Redlich believed that earlier a certain movement upwards was to be remarked. In Germany, very similar studies were conducted by Häfner and Reimann (1970). In spite of the simple explanation which Hollingshead and Redlich had offered, it is easy to see that their research was quoted again and again as proof of discrimination. Scientific discussions finally left the question of lower classes open. Mishler and Scotch (1963), Kohn (1968) and Häfner (1987) have written overviews on the subject.

Friedrich Karl (Frederick C.) Redlich (1910), who emigrated to the USA in 1938 from Vienna, took on special measures with teamwork, with specialists in neighboring disciplines and with young ambitious colleagues. He was president of the Western New England Institute of Psychoanalysis, professor of psychiatry at Yale University and also dean of the medical school there. Redlich was so well-integrated into American Psychiatry that in spite of his background and works written in German, he was barely remembered as German. After the second World War, he personified the in-demand but rare type of combination of clinical university psychiatry and psychoanalysis in the USA. Together with Eugene Bloor Brody he published a book on "Psychotherapy with Schizophrenics" and with Daniel X. Freedman he produced the much used theory book "Theories and Practices of Psychiatry". Both books carried a "point in history" full of calculations and taking into consideration phenomenological and biological aspects.

Leopold Bellak and an Overview of the Problem of Schizophrenia

When Leopold Bellak (1916) listened to the old Wagner Jauregg lectures in Vienna shortly before the second World

War, schizophrenia appeared to be an illness which could soon be understood and controlled. Two decades of research on schizophrenia had produced a large source of literature. However, the subject was far from closed. In 1938, when Bellak first came to the USA, the flood of literature was just beginning there. Ten years later he published his first overview of the schizophrenia literature of the past decade, in which almost 3000 works on schizophrenia appeared. At the same time, the promise to report on the next decade was made. It was strange for such a promise to be kept (Bellak, 1948; Bellak and Benedict, 1958; Bellak and Loeb, 1969; Bellak, 1979). In his first book which still carried the antiquated title "Dementia Praecox", Bellak led the establishment of a research and information center for schizophrenia. This center was established as the NIMH (National Institute for Mental Health) in 1968. This institute, which had a budget of 62 million dollars in 1975, directed 16.1% (almost $10 M) in the same year to research on schizophrenia. One of the publications of the institute is the "Schizophrenia Bulletin" which serves the entire world with continuous information on schizophrenia research and which Bellak had been involved with.

Bellak is in some ways comparable with Redlich. He left Wien (Vienna) in the year of the "union", he is a clinical psychiatrist, schizophrenic researcher, and at the same time psychoanalyst (Spence, 1967). He is a professor of psychiatry at the Einstein College of Medicine in New York and at the same time professor of psychology (psychotherapy) at the New York University. Bellak is also presently considered to have great influence on the American scene, above all in the continuation of his schizophrenia overviews, in which he also outlines European literature which is difficult for the Americans to access because of the language. He is an important mediator for German psychiatry in the USA, which he continuously pays attention to. In his chosen country of habitation, little is left to recognize of his German background. However, in German-speaking countries he is still relatively unknown despite some translations (Bellak and Small, 1972; Bellak, 1981). Bellak is therefore an example of both the benefits and damage of German emigration.

Conclusion and Future Outlook

Looking back, psychiatric immigrants in the USA offer a picture which is varied and not always easily comprehensible. Neither the phenomonologists nor the psychodynamicists found circles of work with people willing to engage in like discussions. The "cultural" currents in America were often difficult for the immigrants to relate with. In spite of this, several psychiatrists succeeded highly. At the beginning of the time of the emigration, shock therapy and psychoanalysis were developing parallel to each other, although shock treatment was fundamentally implemented in psychiatric institutions and psychoanalysis in private institutions and medical practices.

In such a situation, neuroleptics rose up unexpectedly after 1955 in the treatment of schizophrenia. It's meaning was not properly recognized in the USA in the beginning. The tracing of the development of psychopharmaceuticals is not the task of this paper. Heinz Edgar Lehmann, however, should be read on this subject. He first reported in French newspapers in 1953 on the success of chlorpromazine and employed this in the treatment of some of his patients at the Verdun Protestant Hospital in Montreal. With this, Lehmann led the age of psychopharmaceuticologists on the American continent. Reports on his success led to a systematic study of the works of, which fundamentally changed the appearance of psychiatry. Reader's Digest praised Lehmann in 1978 in an essay as the "Healer of the Mind" (Aller, 1978).

Lehmann was born in Berlin in 1911 and, from the age of 5, wanted to be a doctor like his father, Richard Lehmann. By 15 he knew all of Freud's work, because his tutor, who was also a psychologist, introduced him to it. Out of this enthusiasm, Lehmann wanted to be a psychiatrist. In 1929-1935 he studied medicine in Marburg, Freiburg, Wien and Berlin and in 1936 he was promoted over Ferdinand Jahn. His only psychiatric instruction came from Arthur W. Simon and Karl Birnbaum in Berlin in 1937/38, but he was already denied access to their posts, as he was a Jew. In 1937, Lehmann was forced to leave. Because he had waited 1 1/2 years for admittance to the USA, he went to Canada. Without knowledge of the English language, he obtained a visitor's visa, and became a doctor in an institution. Two days later he was employed by Dr.

Porteous of the later Douglas Hospital. At this clinic, Lehmann remained for 39 years. Alone he cared for 600 patients, and still produced a great scientific activity, which earned him a professorship of psychiatry at McGill University for several years. Lehmann never went back to psychoanalysis; however he was a mediator for phenomenological psychiatry, which he had gotten to know through reading. His numerous activities further belong to psychopharmacology.

The new therapy resulted in "new psychiatry" after a time (Maxmen, 1985). This resulted from the necessity for a comparison of results of treatment of psychopharmacology. It was necessary to be able to list psychic changes on a computer. The fundamental philosophical situation offered Hempel's logical empiricism (Schwartz and Wiggins, 1986). It went so far that Hempel himself supplied a "suggestion for the formation of a psychiatric classification" on the demand of the American Psychiatric Association (Saß, 1987). Never had the connection between a philosophical theory and a psychiatric classification been so close. In 1987, Fink, the president of the APA, could assert "DSM III is distanced light years away from DSM II..." and it brings us from a diagnostic world into an atheoretical one. In scientific theory this was recourse to America's English cultural tradition. The philosophical fathers of logical empiricism are all English: Locke, Francis Bacon, and John Stewart Mill. On the psychopathology of "New psychiatry", emigrants could understandably achieve no further contribution. Paradoxically, developments of German psychopathology were still useful in Nazi-Germany; above all Kurt Schneider's symptoms 1 and 2. The result was DSM III (Koehler and Saß, 1984), whose influence on the modern image of schizophrenia is clear: it is translated in 20 languages and 500,000 copies have been sold. Unconnected, in the medical practice in the USA, a psychoanalytically - based idea of schizophrenia lives freely, which is openly much more strongly oriented on therapy than symptomology or nosology.

References

Alexander, F.: Schizophrenic Psychoses. Critical Considerations of the Psychoanalytical Treatment. Arch. Neurol. Psychiat. 26 (1931) 815

Arieti, S.: New View on the Psychology and Psychopathology of Wit and the Comic. Psychiatry 13 (1950) 43-62

Arieti, S.: Interpretation of Schizophrenia. Brunner: New York 1955

Arieti, S.: On Schizophrenia, Phobias, Depression, Psychotherapy, and the Further Shores of Psychiatry. Selected Papers of Silvano Arieti, M.D. Brunner/ Mazel: New York 1978

Arieti, S.: Understanding and Helping the Schizophrenic. A Guide for Family and Friends. Simon and Schuster: New York 1979

Bateson, G.: Language and Psychiatry. Frieda Fromm-Reichmann's Last Project. Editorial Notes. Psychiatry 21 (1958) 96-100

Bateson, G.: Steps to an Ecology of Mind. A Revolutionary Approach to Man's Understanding of Himself. Balantine Books: New York 1972

Bateson, G., D.D. Jackson, J. Haley, J.H. Weakland: Toward a Theory of Schizophrenia. Behavioral Science 1 (1956). G. Bateson: Steps to an Ecology of Mind. A Revolutionary Approach to Man's Understanding of Himself. Balantine Books: New York 1972

Bateson, G., D.D. Jackson, R.D. Laing, Th. Lidz, L.C. Wynne: Schizophrenie und Familie. Suhrkamp: Frankfurt a.M. 1969

Bayle, A.L.J.: Recherches sur les maladies mentales. 1823

Bayle, A.L.J.: Traité des maladies du cerveau et de ses membranes. Paris 1826

Bellak, L. (Ed.): Dementia Praecox; The Past Decade's Work and Present Status: A Review and Evaluation. Grune and Stratton, New York 1948

Bellak, L. (Ed.): Disorders of the Schizophrenic Syndrome. Basic Books, New York 1979

Bellak, L. (Ed.): Was zu viel ist, ist zu viel. Diagnose und Therapie unserer überforderten Gesellschaft. Econ: Düsseldorf- Wien 1981

Bellak, L., and P.K. Benedict (Eds.): The Schizophrenic Syndrome. Logos Press (später Grune and Stratton), New York 1958

Bellak, L. and L. Loeb (Eds.): The Schizophrenic Syndrome. Grune and Stratton, New York 1969

Bellak, L. und S. Small: Kurzpsychotherapie und Notfallpsychotherapie. Suhrkamp, Frankfurt 1972

Bleuler, E.: Dementia praecox oder Gruppe der Schizophrenien. F. Deuticke: Leipzig-Wien 1911

Bleuler, E.: Lehrbuch der Psychiatrie. J. Springer: Berlin 1916, 1983

Bleuler, E.: Textbook of Psychiatry. Authorized English Edition by A.A. Brill, PhB., M.D. Macmillan: New York 1924, 1934

Bruch, H.: Psychotherapy in Schizophrenia. Historical Considerations. In: Strauss, J.S., and M. Bowers (Eds.): The Psychotherapy of Schizophrenia. Plenum, New York 1980

Bryce Boyer, L.: Die psychoanalytische Behandlung Schizophrener. Kindler: München 1976

Burnham, J.C.: Psychoanalysis and American Medicine: 1894-1918. Medicine. Science, and Culture. International Universities Press, New York 1967

Cameron, N.: Individual and Social Factors in the Development of Graphic Symbolization. J. Psychol. 5 (1938) 165-184

Cameron, N.: Reasoning, Regression and Communication in Schizophrenics, 1938

Cameron, N.: A Study of Thinking in Senile Deterioration and Schizophrenic Disorganization. Amer. J. Psychol. 51 (1938) 650-665

Cameron, N.: Deterioration and Regression in Schizophrenic Thinking. J. Abnorm. Soc. Psychol. 34 (1939) 265-270

Cameron, N.: Schizophrenic Thinking in a Problem-Solving Situation. J. Ment. Sci. 85 (1939) 1012-1035

Cameron, N.: Experimental Analysis of Schizophrenic Thinking. In: Kasanin, J.S. (Ed.): Language and Thought in Schizophrenia. W.W. Norton: New York 1964, S. 59-64

Campbell, C.M.: Adolf Meyer. Archives Neurol. Psychiatr. 37 (1937) 715-731

Diethelm, O.: Adolf Meyer. In: K. Kolle (Hg.): Große Nervenärzte. Bd. 2. G. Thieme, Stuttgart 1959, S. 129-138

v. Domarus, E.: Über prälogisches Denken in der Schizophrenie. Zschr. Neurol. Psychiatr. 87 (1923) 84-93

v. Domarus, E.: Beispiele paralogischen Denkens in der Schizophrenie. Zschr. Neurol. Psychiatr. 90 (1924)

v. Domarus, E.: Über die Beziehung des normalen zum schizophrenien Denken. Arch. Psychiatr. 74 (1925) 641-646

v. Domarus, E.: Zur Theorie des schizophrenen Denkens. Zschr. Neurol. Psychiatr. 108 (1927) 703-714

v. Domarus, E.: Über die Halluzinationen der Schizophrenen. Zschr. Neurol. Psychiatr. 112 (1928) 636-638

v. Domarus, E.: Über das Denken der Manischen und Depressiven. Zschr. Neurol. Psychiatr. 112 (1928) 632-635

v. Domarus, E.: Das Denken und seine krankhaften Störungen. Curt Kabitzsch: Leipzig 1929

v. Domarus, E.: The specific Laws of Logic in Schizophrenia. In: Kasanin, J.S. (Ed.): Language and Thought in Schizophrenia. W.W. Norton: New York 1964, S. 104-114

Earles, P.: Institutions for the Insane in Prussia, Austria and Germany. Wood: New York 1854

Ebaugh, R.G.: Adolf Meyer: The Teacher. Archives Neurol. Psychiatr. 37 (1937) 732-741

Eissler, K.R.: Limitations to the Psychotherapy of Schizophrenia. Psychiatry 6 (1943) 381-391

Eissler, K.R.: Remarks on the Psycho-Analysis of Schizophrenia. Int. J. Psychoanal. 32 (1951) 132

Eyrich, M.: Bemerkungen zur Schizophrenielehre und zur verstehenden Psychologie bei Psychosen. Zschr. Neurol. Psychiatr. 127 (1930) 525-533

Faris, R.E.L., and H.W. Dunham: Mental disorders in Urban Areas. University of Chicago Press: Chicago 1939

Federn, E.: Paul Federn: Scholar, Teacher, Pioneer. Complex 3 (1950) 42-46

Federn, P.: Ego Psychology and The Psychoses. Basic Books, New York 1929. Dt. Ichpsychologie und die Psychosen. Huber: Bern-Stuttgart 1956

Federn, P.: Psychoanalysis of Psychoses. Psychiatr. Quart. 12 (1941) 246, 480

Federn, P.: Principles of Psychotherapy in Latent Schizophrenia. Amer.J. Psychother. 1 (1947) 129

Federn, P., and H. Meng: Psychoanalytic Prevention Versus Therapeutic Psychoanalysis. In: Eissler, K. (Ed.): Searchlights on Delinquency. New Psychoanalytic Studies. International Universities Press, New York 1949, S. 26-34

Feuchtersleben, E. Freiherr von: Lehrbuch der ärztlichen Seelenkunde. Als Skizze zu Vorträgen bearbeitet. Carl Gerold: Wien 1845

Freud, S.: Psychoanalytische Bemerkungen über einen autobiographisch beschriebenen Fall von Paranoia (Dementia paranoides). Jahrbuch der Psychoanalyse 3 (1911) 9-69. Gesammelte Werke. Bd. VIII, S. 308. Imago, London 1943

Freud-Jung, Sigmund Freud/ C.G. Jung. Briefwechsel. S. Fischer: Frankfurt 1974

Fromm - Reichmann, F.: Notes on the Treatment of Schizophrenics by Psychoanalytic Psychotherapy. Psychiatry: 11 (1948) 263-273. Auch in: Frieda Fromm-Reichmann: Psychoanalysis and Psychotherapy. The University of Chicago Press: Chicago and London 1959, S. 166. Dt. in neuer Übersetzung in: Paul Matussek (Hg.): Psychotherapie schizophrener Psychosen. Hoffman & Campe: Hamburg 1976, S. 34-52

Fromm-Reichmann, F.: Principles of Intensive Psychotherapy. The University of Chicago Press, Chicago 1950. Dt. Intensive Psychotherapie. Grundzüge und Technik. Hippokrates-Verlag, Stuttgart 1959

Fromm-Reichmann, F.: Psychoanalysis and Psychotherapy. The University of Chicago Press, Chicago 1959. Dt. Psychoanalyse und Psychotherapie. Eine Auswahl aus ihren Schriften. Klett-Cotta: Stuttgart 1976

Gaupp, R.: Zur Psychologie des Massenmordes. J. Springer: Berlin 1914.

Gaupp, R.: Der Fall Wagner. Eine Katamnese. Zschr. Neurol. Psychiatr. 60 (1920) 312

Gaupp, R.: Die dramatische Dichtung eines Paranoikers über den Wahn. Zschr. Neurol. Psychiatr. 69 (1921) 182

Gaupp, R.: Vom dichterischen Schaffen eines Geisteskranken. In: Utitz (Hg.): Jahrbuch der Charaktaerologie 1926

Gaupp, R.: Krankheit und Tod des paranoischen Massenmörders Wagner. Eine Epikrise. Zschr. Neurol. Psychiatr. 163 (1938) 48

Goldstein, K. und Frieda Reichmann: Über die körperlichen Störungen bei der Dementia praecox. (Vorläufige Mitteilung). Neurol. Zbl. 33 (1914) 343-350

Green, Hannah: I Never Promised You a Rose Garden. A Novel. Holt, Rinehart and Winston: New York, Chicago, San Francisco 1964. Dt.: Ich habe dir nie einen Rosengarten versprochen. Bericht einer Heilung. Radius-Verlag: Stuttgart 1973

Griesinger, W.: Die Pathologie und Therapie der psychischen Krankheiten für Ärzte und Studierende. Adolf Krabbe: Stuttgart 1861

Gruhle, H.: Psychologie der Schizophrenie. Julius Springer: Berlin 1929

Gruhle, H.: Die Psychopathologie. In: Wilmans, K. (Hg.): Die Schizophrenie. J. Springer: Berlin 1932

Häfner, H.: Epidemiology of Schizophrenia. In: Häfner, H., W.F. Gattaz, and W. Janzarik (Eds.): Search for the Causes of Schizophrenia. Springer: Berlin - Heidelberg - New York - London - Paris - Tokyo 1987, S. 47-74

Häfner, H. und H. Reimann: Spatial Distribution of Mental Disorders in Manheim. In: Hare, E.H., and J.K. Wing (Eds.): Psychiatric Epidemiology. Oxford University Press: London 1970, S. 341-354

Hoffmann, L.: Grundlagen der Familientherapie. ISKO: Hamburg, 1982

Hollingshead, A.B., and F.C. Redlich: Social Class and Mental Illness. John Wiley: New York 1958

Jacobson, E.: Contribution to the Metapsychology of Psychotic Identifications. J. Amer. Psychoanal. Ass. 2 (1954) 239

Jung, C.G.: Über die Psychologie der Dementia praecox: ein Versuch. 1907. Zit. n. C.G. Jung: Psychogenes der Geisteskrankheiten. Gesammelte Werke. 3. Bd. Walter-Verlag: Olten und Freiburg im Breisgau 1971, S. 1-216

Kahn, E.: Zur Frage des schizophrenen Reaktionstypus. Zschr. Neurol. Psychiatr. 66 (1921) 273-282

Kahn, E.: Schizoid und Schizophrenie im Erbgang. J. Springer: Berlin 1923 a

Kahn, E.: Über Zurechnungsfähigkeit bei Schizophrenen. Mschr. Kriminalpsychol. 14 (1923b) 250-261

Kahn, E.: Versuch einer einheitlichen Gruppierung aller schizophrenen Äußerungsformen des Irreseins. Allg. Zschr. Psychiatr. 84 (1926) 268-274

Kahn, E.: Über die Kombination von manisch-depressivem Irresein und Schizophrenie. Jahreskurse ärztl. Fortbildung, München 17 (1926 b) 18-23

Kahn, E.: Was ist das Schizophrene am Schizophrenen? Mschr. Psychiatr. Neurol. 124 (1952) 328-333

Kahn, E., and L.H. Cohen: Conflict and Integration in Schizophrenic Development. Amer. J. Psychiatr. 89 (1932) 1025-1034

Kahn, E., and L.H. Cohen: Schizophrenia. Pract. libr. Med. Surg. (N.Y.) 9 (1936) 1145-1192

Kant, F.: Ein Beitrag zur Frage schizophrener Symptomenkomplexe (Fall Ernst Müller). Med. Diss. Tübingen 1924

Kant, F.: Über die Kombination reaktiver und charakterologischer mit phasischen und prozeßhaften Faktoren in der paranoischen Wahnbildung. Ein Beitrag zur Frage der "Sensitiven Beziehungs-psychose". Arch. Psychiatr. Nervenkh. 87 (1929) 171-190

Kant, F.: The Structure and Origin of Delusion. 93rd. Annual Meeting of the American Psychiatric Association Pittsburg, Pa. 1937

Kant, F.: Protracted Shocks Occuring During Insulin Shock Therapy and their Treatment. J. Nerv. Ment. Dis. 91 (6) 1940

Kant, F., P.L. Philipps, and R.M. Stolzheise: Problems of Shock Treatment in Schizophrenia. J. Nerv. Ment. Dis. 91 (3) 1940

Kant, O.: Zum Verständnis des schizophrenen Beeinflussungsgefühls. Zschr. Neurol. Psychiatr. 111 (1927a) 417-441

Kant, O.: Beiträge zur Paranoiaforschung. I. Die objektive Realitätsbedeutung des Wahnes. Zschr. Neurol. Psychiatr. 108 (1927b) 625-644

Kant, O.: Beiträge zur Paranoiaforschung. II. Paranoische Haltung in der Gesundheitsbreite. (Vergleichende Analyse, forensischer Ausblick). Zschr. Neurol. Psychiatr. 110 (1927c) 558-579

Kant, O.: Beiträge zur Paranoiaforschung. III. Allgemeine Gedanken zum Wahnproblem. Zschr. Neurol. Psychiatr. 127 (1930) 615-659

Kant, O.: Zur Biologie der Ethik. Psychopathologische Untersuchungen über Schuldgefühl und moralische Idealbildung. Zugleich ein Beitrag zum Wesen des neurotischen Menschen. J. Springer: Wien 1932

Kant, O.: Types and Analyses of Clinical Pictures of Recovered Schizophrenics. Psychiatric Quart. 14 (1940) 676-699

Kant, O.: Study of a Group of Recovered Schizophrenic Patients. Psychiatric Quart. 15 (1941a) 262-283

Kant, O.: A comparative Study of recovered and deteriorated schizophrenic patients. J. Nerv. Ment. Dis. 93 (1941b) 616-624

Kant, O.: The Incidence of Psychoses and Other Mental Abnormalities in the Families of Recovered and Deteriorated Schizophrenic Patients. Psychiat. Quart. 16 (1942) 176-186

Kinross-Wright, V., and E. Kahn: Of Schizophrenia and the Schizophrenic. Amer. J. Psychiatr. 114 (1958) 703-706

Kittel, I.-W.: Arthur Kronfeld on the Occasion of his Hundreth Birthday on January 9th, 1986. Individual Psychology News Letter 34 (1986) 26-28

Kittel, I.-W.: Arthur Kronfeld (1886-1941) Ein früher Wissenschaftstheoretiker der Psychologie und Psychiatrie. Psychologische Rundschau (1) (1986) 41

Koehler, K. und H. Saß (Hg.): Diagnostisches und Statistisches Manual Psychischer Störungen. DSM III. Deutsche Bearbeitung und Einführung. Beltz-Verlag: Weinheim und Basel 1984

Kohn, M.L.: Social Class and Schizophrenia. A Critical Review . In: Rosenthal, D., and S.S. Kety (Eds.): The Transmission of Schizophrenia. Pergamon Press: Oxford 1968

Kraepelin, E.: Psychiatrie. Ein Lehrbuch fur Studierende und Ärzte. Fünfte, vollständig umgearbeitete Auflage. Joh. Ambrosius Barth, Leipzig 1896

Kraepelin, E.: Zur Diagnose und Prognose der Dementia praecox. Allg. Zschr. Psychiatr. 56 (1899) 254-259

Kretschmer, E.: Der sensitive Beziehungswahn. Ein Beitrag zur Paranoiafrage und zur psychiatrischen Charakterlehre. J. Springer: Berlin 1918, 1966

Kronfeld, A.: Das Erleben in einem Fall von katatoner Erregung. Mschr. Psychiat. 35 (1914)

Kronfeld, A.: Über scizophrene Veränderungen des Bewußtseins der Aktivität. Zschr. Neurol. Psychiat. 74 (1922)

Kronfeld, A.: Psychotherapie. Charakterlehre, Psychoanalyse, Hypnose, Psychagogik. J. Springer: Berlin 1923, 1925

Kronfeld, A.: Einige Bemerkungen über Schizophrenia mitis, vornehmlich in psychotherapeutischer Hinsicht. Nervenarzt 1 (1928)

Kronfeld, A.: Über den Wandel des Schizophreniebegriffes. Mschr. Psychiatr. 73 (1929).

Kronfeld, A.: Der Schizophreniebegriff in der französischen Psychiatrie der Gegenwart. Allg. Zschr. Psychiat. 92 (1929)

Kronfeld, A.: Perspektiven der Seelenheilkunde. G. Thieme: Leipzig 1930

Kurianski, J.B., W.E. Deming, and B.J. Gurland: On Trends in the Diagnosis of Schizophrenia. Amer. J. Psychiatry 131 (1974) 402

Laycock, Th.: Mind and brain: or, the correlations of consciousness and organisation; with their applications to philosophy, zoology, physiology, mental pathology, and the practice of medicine. Sutherland & Knox: Edinburgh 1860

Lehmann, H.E.: Die Krankheits - und Heilungslehre des Meiningischen Hofmedicus Ferdinand Jahn. Med. Dis. Berlin 1936

Lehmann, H.E.: Reflections on a Career in Psychiatry. The Canadian Psychiatric Association Bulletin 12 (1980) 14-16

Lehmann, H.E.: Schizophrenia I: Introduction and History. In: Freedman, A.M., and H.I. Kaplan (Eds.): Comprehensive Textbook of Psychiatry. 3rd. ed. Williams & Wilkins: Baltimore 1967, S. 593-598

Lehmann, H.E.: Schizophrenia: History. In: Kaplan, H.I., A.M. Freedman, B.J. Sadock (Eds.): Comprehensive Textbook of Psychiatry. 3rd. ed. Williams & Wilkins: Baltimore/ London 1980, S. 1104-1113. Dt.: Schizophrenie. Geschichte. In: Freedman, A.M., H.I. Kaplan, B.J. Sadock, U.H. Peters (Hg.) Psychiatrie in Praxis und Klinik. Band 1. Schizophrenie, affektive Erkrankungen, Verlust und Trauer. G. Thieme: Stuttgart 1984, S. 20-33

Lehmann, H.E.: Schizophrenia: Clinical Features. In: Kaplan, H.I., A.M. Freedman, B.J. Sadock (Eds.): Comprehensive Textbook of Psychiatry. 3rd. ed. Williams & Wilkins: Baltimore/ London 1980, S. 1153-1192. Dt.: Schizophrenie. Klinisches Bild. In: Freedman, A.M., H.I. Kaplan, B.J. Sadock, U.H. Peters (Hg.) Psychiatrie in Praxis und Klinik. Band 1. Schizophrenie, affektive Erkrankungen, Verlust und Trauer. G. Thieme: Stuttgart 1984, S. 93-142

Lidz, Th.: Adolf Meyer and the Development of American Psychiatry. Amer. J. Psychiat. 123 (1966) 320-332

Lidz, Th.: Adolf Meyer, Psychobiologie et psychiatrie dynamique. Confrontations Psychiatriques 11 (1973) 163-181

Lidz, Th.: Adolf Meyer, International Encyclopedia of the Social Sciences. Macmillan: New York 1968, S. 263-265

Lief, A.: The Commonsense Psychiatry of Dr. Adolf Meyer. Fifty-two Selected Papers. Edited, with Biographical Narrative by Alfred Lief. McGraw-Hill: New York, Toronto, London 1948

Matussek, P. (Hg.): Psychotherapie schizophrener Psychosen. Hoffmann und Campe, Hamburg 1976

Maxmen, J.S.: The New Psychiatry. W. Morrow: New York 1985

Mayer-Gross, W., E. Slater, and M. Roth: Clinical Psychiatry. Ballière, Tindall & Cassel: London 1954, 1970

Meisel, P., and W. Kendrick (Eds.): Bloomsbury/ Freud. The Letters of James and Allix Strachey 1924-1925. Basic Books: New York 1985

Mishler, E.G., and N.A. Scotch: Sociological Factors in the Epidemiology of Schizophrenia, a Review. Psychiatry 26 (1963) 315-351

Oberndorf, C.P.: A History of Psychoanalysis in America. Grune and Stratton, New York,1953

Pélicier, Y.: Consistence du vocabulaire latin de la Folie. Dt. von I.U. Tellenbach: Beständigkeit im Sinngehalt des lateinischen Vokabulars für "La folie" (Verrücktheit). Zschr. Klin. Psychol. Psychother. 30 (1982) 68-76

Pery, H.S.: Psychiatrist of America. The Life of Harry Stack Sullivan. The Belknap Press of Harvard University Press: Cambridge (Mass.) and London 1982

Peters, U.H.: Die Sprache des Schizophrenen. In: Peuser, G. (Hg.): Brennpunkte der Patholinguistik. Fink-Verlag: München 1978

Peters, U.H.: Wortwitz und schizophrene Sprachstoörung - worin besteht der Unterschied? Confinia psychiatr. 22 (1979) 58-64

Peters, U.H.: In Memoriam Erich Sternberg. Nervenarzt 52 (1981) 619-620

Peters, U.H.: Frieda Fromm - Reichmann und die psychoanalytisch orientierte Psychotherapie der Schizophrenie. Fundamenta Psychiatrica 1 (1987) 184-191

Peters, U.H.: Studies in German Romantic Psychiatry. E.T.A. Hoffmann as a Psychiatric Theorist, Justinus Kerner as a Psychiatric Practitioner, London 1988

Pull, C.B., J.D. Guelfi, P. Boyer, M.C. Pull: Les critères diagnotiques en psychiatrie: histoire, état actuel et perspectives d'avenir. Masson: Paris 1986

Redlich, F.C., and E.B. Brody: Psychotherapy with Schizophrenics. International Universities Press: New York 1952

Redlich, F.C., and D.X. Freedman: The Theory and Practice of Psychiatry. Basic Books: New York-London 1966. Dt. Theorie und Praxis der Psychiatrie. 2 Bde. Suhrkamp: Frankfurt 1970. 1974

Sager, Cl.J. und H. Singer Kaplan (Hg.); Edition der Erweiterten deutschen Ausgabe A. Heigl-Evers: Handbuch der Ehe-, Familien- und Gruppentherapie: Kindler: München 1973

Saß, H.: Die Krise der psychiatrischen Diagnostik. Fortschr. Neurol. Psychiatr. 55 (1987) 355-360

Schneider, K.: Die phänomenologische Richtung in der Psychiatrie. Philosophischer Anzeiger 1 (1926) 382-404

Scholz, W.: Charakter, Erlebnis und Wahn-Sinn bei der Paranoia. Eine Untersuchung an Fällen von Eifersuchtswahn. Zschr. Neurol. Psychiatr. 127 (1930) 755-776

Schwartz, M.A., and O. Wiggins: Logical Empiricism and Psychiatric Classification. Comprehensive Psychiatry 27 (1986) 101-114

Shipley, W.C., and F. Kant: The Insulin-Shock and Metrazol Treatments of Schizophrenia, with Emphasis on Psychological Aspects. Psychol. Bulletin 37 (1940) 259-284

Siegler, M., and H. Osmond: Models of Madness, Models of Medicine. Macmillan: New York 1974

Simon, F.B.: Die Grundlagen der systemischen Familientherapie. Nervenarzt 56 (1985) 455-464

Sneshnewski, A.W. (Hg.): Schizophrenie. Multidisziplinäre Untersuchungen VEB G. Thieme: Leipzig 1977

Spence, D.P. (Ed.): The Broad Scope of Psychoanalysis: Selected Papers of Leopold Bellak. Grune and Stratton, New York 1967

Stierlin, H., L.C. Wynne und M. Wirsching (Hg.): Psychotherapie und Sozialtherapie der Schizophrenie. Ein internationaler Überblick. Springer: Berlin - Heidelberg - New York - Tokyo 1985

Waller, A.: Healer of the Mind. Heinz Lehmann's Pioneering Drug Therapy has Enabled Hundreds of Thousands of Mental Patients to Lead More Normal Lives. Readers Digest (1978) 90-94

Wilmans, K. (Hg.): Die Schizophrenie. J. Springer: Berlin 1932

The Concept of Madness in Classic Greece

E. La Croce

Summary: This paper offers a picture of Greek views on madness and its therapy from Homer to Plato.

In Homeric poems the main model of mental illness is that of a sort of possession of the sick man by a demon or divinity. This view is a common pattern in all primitive or archaic cultures. Correlative with it is a magic therapy, and both the Iliad and Odyssey show several instances of treatments of mental diseases by conjuration and prayer.

This conception lasted for a long time, mainly in the popular Greek mind, and connected with it there are certain types of religious cults as Corybantic and Asclepius. During the 5th and 6th centuries B.C. two new models of madness and its treatment are developed. The first is the somatic and natural model characterized by Hippocratic writings, and the second is Plato's philosophical one. While opposing each other neither had a substantial influence on the other.

The historian of psychiatry will be surely more interested on such themes as Socratic heuristic, the Platonic dialectic itself, Aristotle's rhetoric and his interpretation of tragic catharsis. All these subjects, not being directly related with madness therapy, are however concerned with the modern view of it.

OUR CONSIDERATION of the ideas that the ancient Greek had about the consistency, etiology and therapy of mental illness should start, of course, from Homer. The Homeric poems written during the 7th and 8th centuries B.C., constitute the first document of the Greek culture.

The verses of the Iliad and the Odyssey, however, bring the testimony of what the Greek thought was, at the time of 8th century. This is because, as Heraclitus reminds us in the first century A.D.: "From the earliest age, the child's ingenuous spirit that does the first studies, shall be given Homer as food (1)". If the Greek studies Homer during all the ancient time, it should not surprise us that Homeric ideas appear once and twice at many centuries later and remain over everything the popular conception.

The Homeric view of madness, as is obvious, is a function of his vision of man and of his psychic activity. A first approach to it can be obtained through the lightest consideration of the archaeological material. In the most ancient Greek ceramics we find representation of the human figure whose lack of unity, of integrity grabs our attention. The muscles are delineated precisely with emphasis, but legs and arms seem to be separated from the body as if to show the description of the parts rather than its integration of the whole. This has been pointed out by Bruno Snell (2), and seen in the vocabulary of the poet. No single word to designate the body: Soma represents the dead body, Demas the size or physical shape. This is alluded to by a neutral plural word melea, which means "the members".

In parallel, there is not a term to define the personality, as a whole, the itself, or even less psychic structure. The psyche - the soul - is as is known in Homer, is the mere function of life or a residual ghost of the dead body (3). The thymos, all by itself, is something like an organ of the emotional function that on some occasions may keep a dialog with the man, as if it were in some way independent of him.

To summarize, remember the happy expression of H. Frankel (4): The Homeric man is like "an open field of forces". In fact, there are so many examples that describe the mental phenomena as having originated in the exterior of the person.

The same concept of eccentricity is present in the way of considering illness. In the book "The cure with the word in classic antiquity" (5) in 1958 D. Pedro Lain Entralgo catalogued four basic ways of understanding human illness in Homer. They are the traumatic (damage caused by violence in the natural order such as injury, etc.), the ambient, (natural causes, external and not traumatic, such as fatal drugs, mentioned in od 2.329). The last two are the ones that properly relate to illnesses: The punitive way and the demoniac which address the origin of the pain, and which are exclusive one of each other. The first pictured the plague that Apollo sends to the warriors as a punishment for the rape of the daughter of his priest (Il. 1.8 ss). It is about an impure immortal agent perhaps material that penetrates in men. The demoniac way constitutes perhaps the main and generic form which Homer conceives for illness: this is smooth and plainly the possession of the individual by a bad and hostile goddess, a demon. A typical case is the one in Od. 5.394-398; there the "nousos" (sickness) is a demon that chases the person.

In reality, this idea is proper in every archaic mind, and Homer is not the exception; even though this does not necessarily imply a primitive stage of culture. Even the popular language of our time presents similar illustrations when it is said "He is touched" to indicate his madness. According to Dodds (6), the belief in the mental disorder as a product of divine interference "Might have originated in, and been maintained by, the manifestations of the sufferers themselves". It seems to us that this is a way to convert matter, since for the archaic mind every phenomenon which transcends the daily frame of "normality" or her amazing and prominent effect is seen as "divine". Mental illness causes isolated and strange behavior, this is why it is considered to come from an external and divine cause.

Nevertheless, it is necessary to notice that in the Homeric poems there is no allusion to typical cases of complete madness. However, there appears the notion that a rape more or less prolonged by some heroes makes them lose their reason and takes them to wild and irrational behavior. The most notable case is the word "ate". The dictionary of Liddell - Scott - Jones defines it as a "bewilderment, vanity, caused by blindness or delirium sent by gods very often as a punishment for a fury of guilt." It is experienced by Agamemnon when he is forced to give back the raped girl to Apollo, demanding to compensate him with a girl who was owned by Achilles, provoking anger on who caused so much misfortune to Greeks. Then, when he apologized (Il.19.90) saying: "It was not me that caused this act, but Zeus, the destiny and the Erinias that stroll in the darkness; they together put 'ate' in my mind". This type of furious and frantic act proper to warriors, is what Homer designates to the words mania and lyssa, that will be the habits among Greeks to refer to madness.

As is obvious, man will develop therapeutic methods for supernatural sickness which have to have the same magical origin as well. In the case of sickness of natural origin, Homer does not apply the principle of reciprocity. When Ulysses is hurt by a wild boar, Autolycus's sons bind him and stop the hemorrhage with a magical song: (the epode), cfr. od.19.457. The most common method of the Homeric Greeks, and of later ages, was the recitation of formulas accompanied with music. Another variant for sickness is the one of rituals of purification (catharsis) and sacrifices to the offended god who sent the illness as a punishment: the procedures followed (sacrifices, cleansing baths, etc.) the release from the plague of Apollo in the Iliad.

Pedro Lain Entralgo includes also as a therapeutic way "pleasant or suggestive saying" (terpnós logos) which sometimes friends use to help to relieve the pain (eg: the case of Nestor and Patroclo in Ill.15.392). It would be something without a magical procedure. But we believe that in spite of the superlative way the Greeks venerated to the word and trusted the effects, this vehicle of consolation and relief can not be considered as a "therapeutic method".

During the centuries after Homer, there is kept and even developed, the notion of sickness as a demoniac possession or divine punishment as well as the curative practices of supernatural sickness.

In the 6th and 7th centuries (B.C.) the testimonies reveal the eruption of new ways of religious spirituality and a magical conception of the agrarian and popular character is born. This was not visible among the aristocrats of the Homeric world. The mystic of cults of initiation proliferates (eg; cult of Bacchus, orphism, Pythagorism, etc), and diverse religious practices that go from the orgiastic Dionysiac frenzy to the musical cathartic and ascetic of Orphics and Pythagorics will have an important influence in the accidental or intentional therapy of the psychic's pains. As a difference from the epic, the tragic literature of the 5th century displays numerous references to mental illness and shows a great interest in the phenomenon of madness. But the conception of psychic activity detected in the tragedies is different from Homer's. The human soul is not "an open field of forces" where the gods act freely, anymore. It is indicated that agents of behaviors, feelings and thoughts of personages are not divinities but they are in the individual himself, whose psychic life is, without any doubt, as an organization of unity.

But madness continues being something sent by gods. However, this does not constitute a free gift: the personage has it as a result of an internal conflict whose real and transcendental dimension is tied to the human entrail. The symptoms are finely descriptive as we can recognize in the portrait of a melancholic through the bitterness and darkness of Orestes; who is fulfilled by oral-sadistic fantasies. However, the madness of the personage oppressed by Erinyes who chose him for matricide, is illustrated by Euripedes in Orestes with the hallucinations and the delirium proper to paranoia. Euripedes' most interesting work for psychiatry is Las Bacchants where Pentheus's madness, caused by Dionysus and Hercules, kills his family. Also in Sophocles there is a vivid description of a mental disorder in Ajax. This hero is made insane by the goddess of Athens to stop him killing Agamemnon. Hallucinated he kills several animals and guards as if they were his hated enemies. When recovered he falls in to a depressive state and commits suicide.

With reference to the effect of the tragedy on the Athenians that used to observe it during the celebration to honor Dionysus, Aristotle shows in his poetry a phrase whose interpretation has caused a great deal of writing. According to the philosopher, the tragedy, originating in the spectator Phobos and Eleos (fear and compassion), provoke the Catharsis of those passions. (Poet.6,1449b24-31). Because of this, Freud employed the word catharsis to designate one of the processes of the psychoanalytic therapy of groups. That is a fantasy. The objective of the tragedy says Aristotle - is pleasure (hedoné). But this does not prevent the act from having a therapeutic effect in the crowd's emotion. They use another of Aristotle's expressions - only by accident, did the public perceive this function.

No interpretative debate fits here about the famous Aristotle definition (some give to catharsis a sense of moral, others a sense of religion), from Bernays (8), we have the medical interpretation of the term, but take into account the interesting observation of W. Schadewaldt (9): Phobos and Eleos should not be translated for "fear" and "compassion". These terms allude to psychosomatic and elemental effects instead of superior passions. Phobos is what gives you chills or palpitations; Eleos gives you commotion which produces or exacerbates "goose bumps (chicken skin)". The tragedy irritates those conditions homeopathically purifying its excess and then ordering the emotional picture, stretching it and ordering it under a superior meaning.

An interesting testimony about psychotherapeutic practices of mental disorders in the 5th century is found in the theater, not in tragedies but in a comedy of Aristophanes. It is "The Wasps" performed for the first time in 422 B.C. An old Athenian named Philocleon is suffering from madness. His son is looking for the cure and he has given to him several treatments, all unsuccessful; finally he imprisons him. This constitutes a true catalogue of methods used generally at that time for this type of case. Let us quote the text:

> First, he attempted to cure with the word... after to cure with the water... then applied religion and he made him a priest of Cybele. Finally, he took him to Egina and made him rest to cure him in the Asclepius temple. (VV.III-124).

The first therapy mentioned is the persuasion with the word, that of course does not have any technical or systematic character. The second case alludes an ancient ritual of purification that we had found in the Iliad due to the plague sent by Apollo. The last two practices require a little more development.

The priests of Cybele, who were members of the Great Mother Goddess' retinue, made a cult of ecstatic type and allowed frenzy through drums, flutes and other instruments used by highlanders.

The gods who cause mental disorders are mentioned in the Hippolytus by Euripedes (vv. 141 ss) and in the Hippocratic treatise De Morbo Sacro (chap. 1). Greeks had a verb korybantáo, which means "to be under the sacred delirium and have hallucinations". As Dodds (10) pointed out "In the 5th century the priest of Cybele had developed a special ritual for the treatment of madness" and we suppose its orgiastic dance must have produced certain catharsis in a homeopathic way. According to Plato (11) the Priests of Cybele meant to cure the deímata which are "phobias or anxious feelings" according to what Dodds translates (12).

As a testimony to Aristophanes, Greeks who suffered from any kind of illness used to attend the temple of Asclepius, son of Apollo. The key was an incubation treatment, the patients slept in the temple and God sent them a dream. Afterwards followed what moderns call the "secondary elaboration" of the dream the patients told to priests. Then in a "tertiary elaboration" of the dream material they interpreted it and recommended the treatment which consisted not only in sacrifices, purifications, amulets but also as Lloyd (13) says, methods of no magical character such as drugs, diets, phlebotomy, etc (14). The medicines weren't given free and according to some inscriptions in the temple of Epidauro, tell us that a patient who did not pay the fees was punished by the god (15), with marks on his face or a blind man already cured lost his sight back for the same motive (16).

I would be naive in pretending to find here the antecedents of the modern interpretation of dreams. As among Asclepius' followers the sickness is considered a possession or a divine punishment, the same as the priests of Cybele, the most important role of the treatment must have been the diagnosis and surely, the basic objective of inquiring about the dream was to find out what divinity was responsible for the sickness, so it should be cured using all means possible.

Since the 6th century and after, great transformations in the mental categories of the Greeks took place. Simplifying the picture, we could say that the mythic vision of reality was being progressively replaced by other kinds of thoughts of an analytical nature in which consideration of natural processes and intuition about reality is regulated by a rational order, has an important role.

This transformation is shown throughout by certain abandonment of the conception of divine sickness and its treatment with magical actions. However, the ancient religious model still existed combined with the new ideas especially in the ambit of the popular cosmovision.

During the 5th century there was not only mental sickness of divine character but also others of natural causes. Herodotus (17), for instance, detects from Cambises madness that "As a consequence of a corporal sickness", it is not strange that "he had suffered his fantasy and had disordered his sense". It is attributed to Empedocles, a Sicilian philosopher by later testimony of Celio Aureliano (18) that he differentiated a form of sacred madness proceeding from former soul purgaments and the other form as a natural alienation of the mind "from a cause or imperfection of the body".

Plato in a dialog Phaedo (written in 367) shows the same distinction, adding that "madness is a wonderful thing if it has divine origin" (244a and ss). This is a classified in four species: the prophetic, the ritual or telestic, the poetic and the erotic, respectively provoked by Apollo, Dionysus, the Muses and Aphrodite or Eros.

This change of conception is also produced in the therapeutic methods. As Lain Entralgo (19) has observed the word epode, which meant magic psalm - main primitive resource of cure - starts to be used in a metaphoric sense to name the natural effect of the suggestive word.

In a recent work (20), Dr. Bennett Simon catalogues three distinct "models" elaborated by ancient Greeks to present the mental disorders. The first is called by Simon the "poetic model" and corresponds to the conception of madness as possession. The other two - that supplant the first - are the medical (proper of the pseudohippocratic authors) and the philosophical whose first and principal exponent is Plato. We are to refer to this briefly one by one to complete our topic.

The corpus Hippocratium (21) is formed by a quantity of treatments that in antiquity were attributed to the great medical doctor Hippocrates of Cos, contemporary of Socrates, but which pertain to several authors and none can be definitely assigned to Hippocrates. They display certain doctrinaire unity and most of them had been written in the 4th and 5th century possibly.

The corpus (21) helps us with the sacred illness (De Morbo Sacro) and about the Virgins' illness. The first is about epilepsy which was the sacred possession; the second is about hysteria.

The De Morbo Sacro says: Epilepsy "is not more sacred than any other sickness, on the contrary, just as other sicknesses have natural origin this also has a nature (physis) and a definite cause (próphasis)" (22). So, there is no sickness without a natural cause. This statement is accompanied by a severe criticism to "magicians, purificators, vagabonds and charlatans" who deceive patients with enchantments, purifications, baths and diets. The symptoms of epilepsy are described in detail, and the explanation that the cause is defined by the conduction of phlegm which gets blocked then the phlegm penetrates to veins that bring air to the brain. This is seen by the Hippocratic author as the organ of the mental phenomena and the doctor does not hesitate to affirm that madness comes from humidity.

About the Virgins' Illness, the author explains that single women who suffer from mental sickness owe their trouble to retention of blood. He does recommend to get married as soon as possible. In respect to the therapy of mental disorders, there is a diversity of prescriptions that appear at length in the corpus, with emphasis of the administration of potions that are considered to be efficient to eliminate the excess of black and yellow bile.

The Hippocratic consideration about the natural cause of sickness is without any doubt a landmark in the history of scientific medicine. But regarding psychotherapy there is no indication of it in the material written by Hippocrates. It could elaborate an idea badly about the cure of the word because every mental disorder was seen as a product of somatic pain. Moreover, the prescriptions to eliminate the symptoms of mental sickness as Lloyd (23) observes are useless or more than the magical psalms or the purification of the charlatans that the Hippocratic writing condemns.

Finally, let us see the "philosophical model" of madness and its treatment designed in the dialoges of Plato, which are contemporary with the Hippocratics. To the philosopher the human soul (identified with the person) is an organized structure of rational functions, affectives and volitives. Health in consequence is order as is said in Rep. V. "justice", because every part of the soul realized its proper function under direction of the rational faculty (logistikón). The sickness of the soul (nosospsykhés) is interpreted in the Sophist as (227 e and ss) of moral mode and equated with vice or defect. In the Timaus (86b), another dialog of antiquity, two kinds of Illness of the soul are portrayed: The classical mania or madness and the amathia or pathological ignorance, that seems to correspond to mental retardation.

In Plato we find the exact contrast to the Hippocratic vision. The health of the soul is the condition of the health of the body (24) and the soul is healthy when it has "sophrosyne" (25), which means moderation, temperance, hierarchical harmony in which senses, lustful wishes, irascible appetite are placed under the direction of that spiritual part of the soul which "is not from this world" and which is naturally turned over to the contemplation of the spiritual ambit of ideas.

The Platonic dialectic, heiress of that heuristic or the "art of breaking of concepts" attributed to his master Socrates, constitutes the suitable method of conquering the health of the soul.

We can talk truly about a real "cure with the word". However, it is precise to recognize that very little of what we now say that the term psychotherapy means is present in Plato. According to his criteria "most of men are crazy" (26), because the health of the soul is a goal only reachable by the philosopher and his "psychotherapy" a philosophical process of spiritual conversion. It happens that for Plato "normality" was not only the good adjustment to society or the absence of psychopathologic symptoms, but also the exact realization of the man, metaphysical enterprise.

According to what we have seen, the substitutive models of mental sickness as a divine possession - Hippocrates' and Plato's - are absolutely opposed, and neither of them anticipates the perspective which today faces the suspect of madness, some because of its excessive somatism and the other because it is referring to another order of things. No influence seems to have surfaced among themselves and the Olympians a mutual ignorance that separates them and made impossible any type of synthesis.

The history writers of psychiatry for certain will experience major interest, respect for the treatment of psychic pain. In themes such as Socratic heuristic, the same Platonic dialectic, the rhetoric of Aristotle or the interpretation of the tragic catharsis according to him, all those affairs were not referred directly to the treatment of madness, but which may by accident have something to do with it.

References

1. All Hom. I.

2. cfr. Die Entdeckung des Geistes. Studien zur Entstehung des europäischen Denkens bei den Griechen, Hamburg 1946 (hay trad. esp.)

3. El primer estudio importante de la psicología en Homero está en la célebre obra de E. Rohde, Psyche, Freiburg 1898 (hay trad. esp.). Sobre la evolución del tratamiento del tema desde entonces, cfr. W. Jaeger, La teologia de los primeros filósofos griegos (trad. J. Gaos), México 1952, cap. V. y C. Eggers Lan, La idea de alma en Homero (mimeogr.). Bs. Aires, 1968.

4. Dichtung und Philosophie des frühen Griechentums, München 1962. cfr. pp. 80 ss.

5. Madrid 1958, cfr. cap. 1.

6. The Greeks and the Irrational, Boston 1951, p. 66. Hay trad. esp.

7. A Greek-English Lexicon, 9 th. ed., Oxford 1940, repr. 1961, s.v. ate.

8 Zwei Abhandlungen über die Aristotelische Theorie des Drama, Berlin 1880. Cfr. la obra de Else, Aristotle's Poetics: The Argument, Cambridge (Mass.) 1967.

9. Cfr. su. artículo en Hermes 83.

10. op. cit. p. 77.

11. Leyes 790e.

12. op. cit. p. 78

13. Magic, Reason and Experience. Cambridge 1979, p. 45.

14. Esto último según Aelio Aureliano, Or. XLVIII. 47.

15. Insc. Gr. IV 951-953.

16. Citadas por Lloyd en op. cit. p. 46 n. 202.

17. Hist. 3.33.

18. Morb. Chron. I, 5.25. Corresponde a Diels-Kranz 31A98.

19. op. cit. p. 91 ss.

20. Mind and Madness in Ancient Greece, London 1978.

21. Publicado por E. Littré, Hippocrate, Oeuvres complétes, Paris, 1849.

22. cap. 2 par. 2.

23. cfr. op. cit. p. 49.

24. cfr. Cárm. 156d-157a.

25. Cárm. 159b.

26. La frase es de Simon, op. cit. p. 170.

From Insane Poor to Poor Insane: An Examination of the Insane and Insanity in Baroque Rome

C. Kläui

Summary: The author describes the evolution of the Hospitale delli poveri forestieri e Pazzi in Rome from 1561 to 1635. The hospital had been founded by a lay brotherhood in order to house needy foreigners, mainly poor pilgrims to Rome. It also received the needy mentally ill. In the course of time it was changed into an asylum exclusively for the mentally deranged. In that respect, it became the first lunatic asylum in Italy. The various rules of the house show the changing attitudes in the care of the poor and in handling the mentally ill.

IN THE FOLLOWING research paper, the process of the first institutionalization of Rome's mental health care, which was installed in the middle of the 16th century, will be traced. Special consideration will be given to related changes in the societal position of mental patients, and to the perception of insanity itself. A great restructuring of a socioeconomic nature (growing urban poverty), an ideological kind (the counterreformation and beginning of the Baroque), and important changes in systems of health care will be examined. We have examined the development of the "Hospitale delli poveri forestieri e Pazzi" which was to become the first Italian mental institution, investigated all traceable (only partly published) sources for the period between 1561 and 1635; with the background of an analysis of urban social structure and the developments in public assistance methods. On this subject, we made use of numerous contemporary descriptions of the "religious and charitable" institutions, and we consulted decrees on poor and social policies, different hospital regulations, reports of apostolical visits, and further various sources. The partly Latin, partly Italian manuscripts and printed sources have been taken from the following places: Archivio segreto del Vaticano (ASV); Biblioteca apostolica del Vaticano (BAV); Archivio dell'Ospedale di S. Maria della Pietà (ASMP); Archivio di Stato di Roma (ASR).

Further, we will support our findings with new works on the historical investigation of types of assistance available in Rome at the time, and the poverty problem in Rome and other parts of Europe. Important information on the economic and social life of Rome was obtained from the extensive work of J. Delumeau. Among the little work available on the origin of Rome's first mental institutions, the "Studi sulla pazzia nella provincia di Roma" by A. Gianelli should be especially mentioned as an important source.

A remark should be made regarding the use of language. In the historical deficiency of comprehensive developments and clearness of Latin and Italian texts, we employ colloquial language concepts such as "insane", "insanity", and "craziness" without implying a modern psychiatric terminology. This also applies to the concepts of "poor" and "poverty", in social, economic, and also moral terms; they are contained in a changing mixted ratio. Through the alteration of this mixed ratio, these concepts, in regards to the time period, suffer a shift in meaning, which must be taken into consideration in order to gain an adequate understanding of the subject.

I. From Poor Asylums to Mental Hospitals

1. 1563- The new "Hospital for Poor Foreigners and the Insane"

> It is given that the fulfillment and completion of a godly law contains God, our Lord, and the loving of our neighbour, and our brothers, and that no one can boast of loving God (whom no one sees), if he does not first love and do good to his neighbour (who is right before his eyes). Love then means nothing other than doing good; in this way one loves. From here, it follows that one who desires to fulfill the law and serve our God, and sees the miserable who lie in the streets and die of cold, must lend their mercy with one or two beds in a small house, in order to help these poor beings.

This is how the "decree, statute, and constitution of the company of Madonna of the Pietà of Houses or Hospitals of poor foreigners and the insane in the exalted city of Rome" begins (1563). This document contains a summary of the genesis of hospitals and their first statutes. It is one of the founding documents of an institution which would a decade later become the first mental asylum of Rome.(1)

The amateurness of this merciful institution offered it's hospitality to the mentioned "poor", and "also to foreigners, who find no lodging, who are starving, who know nothing, and know not which way to turn."(2) Later, as a historical glance backwards tells us, this grand hospital would continue to admit and receive mental patients:

> Currently in Rome there exists no house or hospital for those insane and robbed of reason, and that many of such a kind, distressed people found naked, barefoot, and without direction, who are dying of cold and other things, without help for their freezing bodies, were all taken into the above named hospital for lodging. In this hospital they should be guided and nourished with all they need and provided with remedies when necessary.(3)

In 1563, the hospital also served those poor who were helpless, abandoned, and shelterless, who had no one to support them, and who would perish from cold and hunger. Whether they were foreigners entering the city without reference, or poor who had been rendered helpless by bodily weakness, or the insane wandering naked and barefoot through the city; their misery made them all equal and they therefore deserved to equally find a bed and warm food in the hospital.

Beggars, idlers and vagabonds were not to be admitted, who, in opposition to those finding a way open to a hospital place, were seen as "holding to life as a performance."(4) Such people were to accept human destiny, which God granted to Adam with the words "by the sweat of your face shall you eat your bread, until you again become part of the earth you came from."

Treatment in the Hospital

The documents permit us an insight as to what happened to poor staying in the hospital. First, known rituals from pilgrim care, such as foot washing and body care, with biblical directions on foot washing were promoted (Johannes 13, 1, 20). In this way, the poor became admonished and instructed in the charity doctrines and religion, as many pious and merciful directions of the time obliged them.(5)

Treatment in the hospitals was fundamentally equal for all. The insane were given no special consideration.(6) That the insane were given "medicaments, when necessary", appears nevertheless to speak of some differential treatment. However, this is not particularly valid, if one considers that medical supply provisions (salves, oils, bandages, etc.) are part of customary duties, and there is no talk of application of other specific medications.

The Poor Insane

In 1561, a papal decree was published - the oldest available document of the hospital of S. Maria della Pietà, - licensing the brotherhood "in the name of poor foreigners" (pauperum advenarum); which gave them the right to dictate the statutes/ articles on hand from 1563.(7) The Latin text of the decree reveals observations of social misery suffered by the poor and homeless, and those "deprived of reason" similar to those found in the statutes. In both texts, the insane are designated with no further specification than "robbed of reason" ("mentis inopes qui rationis orbati iudico" which is called "privi d'intaletto" in the decree) no further evidence on insane beings is found, save a single mentioning of "madness".(8)

As to what constitutes the insanity of the insane, no differing sensibilities are considered. Far more detailed and comprehensive on the other hand, are the descriptions of what characterized the insane, in order to be hospitalized: poverty, homelessness, helplessness, passing out from cold and hunger. These are special conditions in which the insane could in no way be differentiated from other poor finding accommodation in the hospital. Rather, they were all considered in general, as the same. Because of a general social standing, all poor could equally find lodging in the hospital. In the admissions policy of "the hospital of foreigners and the insane", insanity was not the primary consideration according to the mentioned documents, but rather, poverty and homelessness. Whatever the "deficiency of reason" meant remains nebulous. It will suffice that any individual to whom the concepts "matti" or "pazzi"(9) or "dementi" could be in some way connected. Only in vague and uncertain ways were the insane also seen as ill; what one can conclude from this is that a "recovery" would be deemed possible.(10) What does come across precisely is these people's material and physical situation of need. What the insane received in terms of mercifulness, provisions, and supplies, was not determined by their insanity, but by their material life situation. Subject to hospital admission was not the figure of the insane, who could be poor, but the figure of the poor, who could be insane.

2. 1592: Changes and Crises in the Structure of the Hospital

From the handwritten books of the hospital administration, found in the archives of the roman mental hospital, S. Maria della Pietà, we can conclude that around 1580, references to "poor foreigners" disappear.(11) Only the "pazzi", "pazzarelli", or "poveri pazzi"; the "insane" continue to be mentioned. A list from June 1574 referring only to the insane contains 27 madmen and 22 madwomen.(12) 1592 listings show 24 men and 22 women admitted to the hospital.(13) Further on in the document, however, the patients are also labeled homeless, helpless and ill. (In 1635 this poverty criterion will be missing, as we will see: insanity will replace poverty as a definitive characteristic.)

In 1592, Pope Clemens VIII arranged a visit to all churches and religious institutes in Rome, on the occasion of his entrance to office. From four short manuscripts it is clear that measures taken in hospitals were inspired by social and church policies.(14)

In these texts, the hospital is depicted as a deficient and badly run operation. New aims are outlined to be placed under a functioning administration.

What are the critical points? The company was falling in on itself since the founding of the hospital. No further worries were directed towards the institution "whether out of mercy or bureaucratic duty." The 15 employees designated to 46 insane patients could no longer carry out their work "as form and guidance were lacking". Because of the cramped quarters and filth caused by the sick, an awful stink was emitted, harming not only the sick themselves, but also the entire neighborhood. Indeed, beds for the sick and the employees were sufficiently equipped with mattresses, linen and covers; as well, the kitchen had necessary utensils, but supplies of all types: wine, bread, wood and oil were lacking. An orderly medical provision/ supply gave so little in the way of medicaments that the demands on the hospital were inevitably not met, and the poor were left to die in misery.(15)

This was the description of the sad state of the hospital. The original concepts seemed to have failed and the hospital was in a state of neglect and destruction. The interest of the papal administration seemed negligible. The cardinal, who was to have taken over protection of the hospital, did not act. Papal coffers offered no financial support.

In the texts of 1592, the insane are no longer described with the same terms as in 1563. Indeed, poverty remained an important characteristic for apostolic figures, but social concerns were no longer valid. The insane were not only homeless, helpless and poverty stricken as in 1563, but also segregated by their insanity. They were no longer excluded and necessarily poor.(16) No longer unequivocally defined through their social position, they were also not, however, clearly defined through insanity itself. Frequently, they were merely classified as ill. One text suggested that the hospital should resign as a self-standing institution, and that the insane should be housed in a medical hospital in Rome; this is an implied submission of insanity as a medical concept of disease. Therefore the papal administration did not follow this suggestion. Their negligible interest seems to have stopped altogether, and nothing appears to have moved or changed in the hospital. What of the insane now? Poor, but self-defined through their insanity? Observations of their differences from other poor began to increase, and a clearer conception of what they were began to manifest itself.

3. 1635: A Mental House Resolves Itself

With the statute reforms of 1635, the crisis was less severe. Cardinal Francesco Barberini, who signed the new statutes (17), as protector of the hospital, had a direct knowledge of problems and reproaches, as well as being a representative of the papal administration with considerable sociopolitical foresight.

In these statutes, the insane were given a face for the first time, where the features and tendencies of insanity itself were brought to expression, if still in a coarse and rudimentary form. The occupants of the reformed hospital of S. Maria della Pietà were for the first time decisively insane. They could be homeless and poor, one would like to characterize them as sick, but only a very certain manifestation of insanity made a person a potential subject for the hospital. It is therefore not astounding that in the statutes of 1635 we find sufficient material to give us a representation of an average hospital day of an insane occupant. This new reception of insanity presented a practical problem, for treatment guidelines had to be drawn up.

Nevertheless, the statutes did not have the insane as their object, but rather the hospital. They regulated the administration, which was led as exercises of an independent functioner. Descriptions of employee's duties are found, containing important observations on the living situation of insane patients.

The statutes of 1635 differentiate themselves in tone, with their certainty of declarations and secure aims; the figure of the insane is outlined, contrary to the statutes of 1563. The religious - theological elements of the text are kept to a minimum and a pragmatic - administrative tone is prevalent.

The Poor Insane

The idea that the insane were fundamentally poor and homeless was decreasing in the new statutes. The new question posed was how far the insane inflicted "great damage to their fellow neighbors", that is to say, visible, active, conclusive insanity. Namely, "continual unreasonable screaming, or the throwing away of objects and similar behavior". Not every "negligible mental disorder" was valid as insanity; that is to say, admission criteria. Those who were "only a little stupid, or occasionally off" would not be accepted.(18)

There were two fundamentally new differentiating criteria to the mental institution of 1635, relative to its acceptance policies. First was necessary hospitalization for insane disturbing their surroundings. Hospitalization was, for a large part, based on protection of the environment; however, damage was no more closely defined than this. Secondly, any person inflicting damage on their surroundings, excluding hospital patients, were considered insane. Action is the connecting link of both criteria and the focus of sensitivity. A conclusive criteria for insanity is essential for the insane being and causing damage to one's neighbors comprises exactly this.

With this, the 1563 differentiation of poor vs. non-poor disappeared, and instead the insane were separated from the sane. At this point, only a scant half of the patients were not in a situation to answer for their own subsistence.(19)

To these people, no bill was sent. Those who could pay their way would be better treated than those who couldn't.(20) Books from the hospital and reports of apostolic visits depict this better than ever.

Vis a vis the statutes of 1563 one finds a two-fold shifting of attention: in 1563 detailed explanations of the misery of homeless and helpless poor seeking protection are given as motives on which admissions were founded; these points are no longer outlined in 1635. The protection of surroundings was then rendered prominent as the function of the hospital. Secondary, in 1563, only a very general and restricted definition of insanity as "deficiency of reason" was given; this was however bound to a social level with the conditions of homelessness and poverty. By 1635 a description as to what insanity means was clearly laid out. The question as to how an insane being expressed himself in his behavior, is central ("l'esser pazzo s'intende che faccia pazzia formali"). The expressions of insane conduct are what constituted troublesome social problems. This is also apparent in the primitive "diagnostic" criteria which lead to an applicant's acceptance.

However, this still does not imply a medical system. A doctor was not required to ascertain whether a patient should be admitted or not.(21) A doctor was immediately called, however, if a patient required purgative treatments; in other words, was "sick" (meaning either surgically or medically). The function of insanity itself had little to do with measures the hospital implemented regarding the insane. At the time, existing knowledge of "mental illness" was not represented. The care of the insane remained a social, rather than a medical, problem.

The Insane in the Mental Institution

The hospital of 1635 was a closed institution. The insane could not be let out alone, but by twos in the custody of a guard, under observation. "Difficult degrees" of insanity took away the right to move freely in the institution; they were put in rooms with ankles bound, chained to beds, or put in a "straw room", like a cell, with an idea given to raving madness or frenzy.(22)

The "mastro de pazzi" conducted an inspection over all types of accommodation "to make those admitted afraid; fear is what most lead and keep the place quiet." The position of this office obviously demands a personality which was beautifully described:

> It is of great importance that this post is exercised with mercifulness and discretion. If one does not exercise proper caution and great attention, and the overseer is not exceedingly tactful and composed, grave errors will occur quickly; the poor will be mistreated and excessively beaten, or too strongly held in straw or other places. However, it is also most dangerous and leads to failure if the named master is powerless and weak, and does not have enough understanding of carefulness to make them afraid. (23)

Special attention was given to the separation of males and females.(24)

The dangerousness of the insane is taken as a theme in application to their treatment in the hospital:

> An insane person must not be allowed to enter the kitchen, wardrobe, or supply room. There should be no wood, iron, or other things which could cause damage left in the institution. No lights shall be lit where the insane are; in winter they shall also eat their evening meal by daylight. Hot pans, when necessary in winter, shall be left covered with narrow, horizontal iron bars, far from fire. In the institution, absolutely no glass shall be used, only in clay plates, tin glasses and clay keys. (25)

Whether threats were thought to be inflicted on others or the self is not clear.

This dangerousness of the insane, their potential damaging to "fellow man" was a criterion not yet apparent in the language of 1563; now insanity posits and specifically characterizes the insane. The discovery of insanity as an institutional problem is it's recognition as a social danger. In 1563, insanity wore the clothing of the helpless poor; now it wears the garments of social danger. Whether it manifested itself as raving or stupid, marked strong or weak; it was always a social entity of a special type. The mental institution of 1635 removed the insane from the great mass of poor, and installed them as a special group. Their poverty was no longer grounded on the material; it is sure that they remained poor in a moral sense. The insane poor had become the poor insane.(26)

II. The Socio-Political Context

1. Poverty in Rome

Now that we have seen the genesis of the first Italian institution, and with it the depiction of a new perception of the insane and their insanity, we will now examine the essential background leading to a different development of the first institutionalized core of the insane.(27)

In 1527, the royal troops of Karl V invaded papal Rome. The mass murder and plundering coming with the event (hence the name "Sacco di Roma") carries important implications. Sacco depopulated the city in which almost 30,000 people were living. The number of inhabitants then climbed from 1700 to 150,000. Many factors were involved in this quite unlinear population development: bad harvesting with grain shortages, the unsolved problem of the Pontinism swamp, the flooding of the Tiber, migration of the plagues, malaria and typhus epidemics.

This dynamic population development along with uncertain economic changes affecting all of Europe, and poverty-stricken land owners swarming into the city in masses, were also particulars.

In the 16th and 17th century, the Roman economy was predominated by food stuffs and textiles. Artisan production was strong; therefore productive branches did not expand, in contrast to other important Italian cities. The building sector devoured a lot of money, however it produced no exportable product. Attempts of several popes to widen the productive base of industry had failed, in resistance from the feudal aristocracy and tradition oriented, as well as the economic freedom of feared artisan's guilds.

The situation of poorer societal stratas deteriorated over the century after the Sacco di Roma. From the second half of the 16th century on, the poor part of Rome's population clearly increased, both absolutely and relatively. It is nevertheless difficult to create a clear picture of the dimensions of poverty with no quantitative declarations available. There was poverty in the streets: beggars, loafers, vagabonds, thieves, prostitutes were to be found in hospitals, cloisters and prisons.(28) Poverty was poorly concealed in circles of underpaid, badly equipped service workers, and opportunity seekers.

In 1555, the "Avvisi di Roma" regularly reported difficulties with food supplies. With the famine of the following year, farmers were driven into the city without accommodation to join the numbers of the hungry urban poor. Grain supplies from surrounding regions of Rome were not extensive enough; corn supplies from other areas of Italy became increasingly necessary. This turned into a great social crisis. Above all, however, the papal administration succeeded in preventing great social conflict like in the Neapel Masaniellos or the Palermo hunger revolts, at the cost of the interior and other church states.

2. The Roman Care of the Poor and Sick

The small city which Rome became after Sacco could rely on a pre-built hospital system and a good system of charity and alms. Both had their roots in the middle ages. A quantitative measure of the conditions is hard to get, but one can be sure that sick-assistantship from 1527 was well endowed. The hospitals pass as modern, and were praised by outside visitors, among them Martin Luther.

In open hospitals, like everywhere, the poor were predominantly placed. The rich were mainly treated at home; doctors and surgeons were not lacking to them, however, they only worked in small areas of the hospitals.

Bad hygiene and living conditions, poor nourishment and body care, plagues and other hospital epidemics were some of the things amounting to occupants being predominantly poor. General historical roots of hospitals were as provisions for the poor, foreign and pilgrim accommodations, and care-related duties. Hospitals at the beginning of the 16th century had often not yet stopped serving these functions.

Besides alms, the poor had a long and stable history of private charity at their disposal. Aid was an integral component of the every-day life of the rich, and in special masses, the pope himself could count on the charity of the church leaders.

The bearers of charity and care in Rome were friars, lay-brother societies, artisan corporations and representatives of several nations. The rising of central operations was scarce, and restricted to emergency situations such as plagues. What took over were repressions such as city expulsions of vagabonds and foreign beggars; compulsory admittance to hospitals/ military hospitals in times of hunger and epidemic threats.

After the socio-economic crisis in the middle of the sixteenth century, an uncontrolled growth came in manifold institutions, after the previous pluralistic system. Without centralized planning, projects were undertaken where a need was recognized. The founding history of S. Maria dell Pietà is typical for this time. Repressive measures predominated since the time of the pontificate Paul IV (1555-1599). The expulsion of bandits, vagabonds, unemployed, and gypsies took place; the banning of begging from churches and a whole set of other restrictive precautions were put into place "for the betterment" of morality. A good one third of the population were in need of some kind of solution. The risk of social tensions and revolts was high, and had to be prevented.

The whole of Europe was shaken by the problem of poverty and erratic social transformations - this is the time of the council of Trent for the Catholic church, and the beginning of the counterreformation - discussions on the theme of poverty were arising; Luther Erasmus and Ludovico Vives belong to this time. The central points of the debate were: assistantship to the lay brother, centralization under city (later state) sovereignty. The development of differentiating criteria for those able to work, native vs. foreign, genuine vs. false, support - worthy vs. non support-worthy, the poor in connection with forced work and back-up measures, and expulsion strategies.

Attempts to implement programs were first evident in England, and then Holland and Germany, with work houses and education houses as an expression of new policies.

The calling for new forms of intervention was audible in the coming to a head of the poverty problem and a climate of increasing unrest. The papal administration had to open up it's assets - still to be revised at Trent - the speaking against tradition was not rare in the Reformation.

> Evidently, - Simoncelli wrote, - necessity began to pave the way for an organized and open concept of containment of the poverty

> phenomenon, which showed a new face, more aggressive than that of the Renaissance which was good-natured, such as the appearance of begging in the comedies of Aretino. It is the 'new poor', who are frightened perhaps for the first time by the city authorities, who were used to treating and solving the entire question of poverty and begging with wide philanthropic interventions; with concepts which are evidently no longer sufficient to keep the social and political phenomenon within acceptable borders. (29)

Shifting in central ideas came first under Gregory XIII (1572-1585), who in 1581 wanted to accommodate all beggars in Rome in a former Dominican cloister on the Via Appia. The experiment failed after 2 years, the main reason being not so much opposition from poor to being enclosed by force, but more because of poor financial support of the project.

A renewed enclosure of the poor began in 1587 under Sixtus V, who founded the "Hospedale de' poveri mendicanti di San Sisto" in the framework of measures to fight against poverty and hunger. In 1591, more than 2000 poor were locked up and contained, more than 2% of the city's population.

Because of a decrease in donations to San Sisto after the death of Sixtus V, several years followed of successive decay to this instrument of centralist policies. Beggars, who had no other way of making their living, were forbidden begging licenses. Demands for assistanceship were again increasing.

In resistance, a great number of the bearers of assistance, through specialized privately organized institutions, who found their existence threatened by centralized policies and a transferring of papal monies, found a principal reason for the failure of large-scale internment campaigns.(30)

The social problems remained in a state of urgency. Only a system of compromise between the leading wealthy stratas and corporations, taking into consideration the necessity of an efficient assistance policy in the form of a lenient central control, could successfully prevail.

> The assistance system which was constructed with the beginning of the pontificate of Clemens VIII, - writes Simoncelli, - appears to actually be a practical interim solution between the old, philanthropic, and in economic hindsight, self-sufficient system of the Renaissance, and a state centralized system like Sixtus V. had begun. (31)

The essential lines of development of Roman assistance methods of the 17th century were already indicated by the end of the 16th century. "The 17th century is innovative; at best it perfected a system; at least in this way it was a time-axis of the century."(32)

Assistance methods experienced a change, with true developments of the 17th century, such as enforced polycentralization of emerging organizations and essential responsibility for these further developments. It was these institutions, whose activities were distinguished by precise rules, by clear and strict forms of organization, and by high levels of efficiency. It was especially the Fatebenefratelli who enforced authoritative health methods in Rome and all of Italy. Their influence on the statute reforms of 1635 must not be overlooked. The merciful brothers, typical of the 17th century, also undertook pioneer duties of the care of the insane: they were involved in several hospitals and "maisons de force" during the "great imprisonment" (Foucault) in France under Louis XIV. In the 18th century, they also engaged in Italian mental health care, establishing a modern-type lunatic asylum on the island of San Servolo, near Venice. In the 19th century they participated .in the boom of newly established mental asylums in Italy.

Conclusions

In the transition from the 16th to 17th century, a new face appeared among the population of Rome. The societal character mask of the "insane" continued as an amorphous mass of poor. As the above work portrayed changes in assistance measures and in the "mental house" itself, so did a social conception of insanity separate itself through self-defined criteria. It was the institution for the insane which first gave rise to this new identity.

Of course, here we do not have the birth of insanity, or it's perception before us. The contemporary Italian doctors had a different diagnostic repertoire of "mental diseases" than representatives of institutional care of the insane. Mental patient care itself was naturally not first developed in the asylum. The insane were originally treated in a more or less repressive fashion.

However, the specific social meaning given to insanity was new. It was not a matter of course, unrelated to time, that the insane patient necessarily implied a professional, specialized, institutionalized "answer", as is this answer, which created a certain societal role for the insane, and which introduced a development, which validates the care of the insane to the present day. It is interesting to ask why, and under what conditions the care of the insane developed.

We have tried to answer this question on the example of Rome, and we are pushed on the paradox of hard facts, that the formation of insane organizations as at the most, had little to do with insanity. The installing of the insane in Rome's first "mental institution" was closely dependent on their social situation of homeless poor. Their material poverty was a repeated factor. The paradox is understood if one takes into consideration development tendencies in assistance methods of the time, and uneven changes in Rome's structure - especially through a serious increase in poverty in connection with the formation of the general European phenomenon of pauperism. New concepts of poor policies were primarily built on the poor in an ideological-political process new to make groupings of support-worthy sick and non-support worthy, work-capable poor. At the same time, establishments for the poor and sick were differentiated and separated. Hospitals of the middle ages which housed all needy, regardless of their specific situations, were transformed slowly with new criteria of care, as in special establishments with special instructions for the poor; they contained this special new group of "unworthy" poor of referred-to repression policies. In this process, the hospital Santa Maria della Pietà developed as an institution with special characteristics for a defined group of needy. The new statutes of 1635 carry the mark of the leading hospital statutes, of the "merciful brothers and employees of San Camillo de Lellis, der Ministri degl'infermi." The insane were in an institution to become a defined group through their insanity, who had lost their social identity of poverty. The poverty of the insane remained linguistically contained, but was transferred from a socioeconomic to a moral concept.

One could try to establish a speculative connection between the process which made the insane poor into poor insane, and the new strategies which differentiated genuine poorness from false; meaning the subjectivity of the idea of intention: with it a group of poor can be defined as "false" and "unworthy" and as the object of a new strategy of discipline. This must have separated a logical ideological operation of "support-worthy" and "valid" poor. Contemporary demands on the poor to be pious and devoted, and to raise will to work, assume the separation of each; the insane would lose their strength through this polemic of absurdity.

The pragmatic correlation of this operation is given in the hospital and obvious cases of insane. Even if the care of the insane was in reality hardly effective, many insane gave up their desolate destinies, and if they were neglected in instances for a long time, - as we can gather from the texts of 1592, the mere presence of insane asylums has a fundamental meaning in the recognition of the insane as special cases. Moving into the 18th century the insane were of central interest, when a new societal dynamic of integration created new potential forms of refusal. For the first time, an important increase in the number of insane asylums and an increase in their direct sociopolitical applications took place.

Even if medical care in the 16th and 17th centuries found it's way in the traditional family path, the origin of the stationary institutional treatment was marked by charging societal behaviour towards insanity and the insane. In the disciplinization of poverty the separation of insanity as a deficiency of reason and free will was achieved. This separation process remains characteristic of the social relations to insanity up to the present day. As far as we can recognize the roots of modern day organizations for the insane, different components and the disciplinization of insanity itself is still missing.❧

References and Notes

1. Ordini, Statuti, & Constitutioni della Compagnia della Madonna della Pietà della Casa, over Hospitale delli Poveri forestieri, & Pazzi, dell'Alma Città di Roma, Rom 1563. ASV, Arm. IV, t. 9, p. 92 r- 99 v, p. 92 v.

2. op.cit., p. 92v. Der Begriff "Hospital" bedeutet im 16. Jahrhundert primär "Hospiz", kann aber auch die Bedeutung "Krankenhaus" haben.

3. op.cit., p. 94v, 95r.

4. op.cit., p. 94v, und 95r.

5. op.cit., p. 94v.

6. Zwar wird die dauernde Präsenz einer Wache explizit nur für die Irren gefordert, doch ergibt sich aus den Aufgaben, die sie zu erfüllen hat, kein Hinweis auf Charakteristika, die die Irren von den übrigen untergebrachten Armen unterscheiden würden. Auch fehlt jeder Hinweis auf eine gesonderte Unterbringung der Irren. In diesem Zusammenhang ist auch interessant, daß die hygienischen Maßnahmen im Text einzig auf die armen Fremden bezogen werden, was natürlich, wollte man daraus schließen, daß die andern Gruppen davon ausgeschlossen sind, keinen Sinn ergäbe.

7. Bulle von Pius IV. "Illius qui pro dominici", 11.9.1561, zit. nach: Gianelli, A.: Studi sulla pazzia nella provincia di Roma, Rom 1905, p. 68-72.

8. Ordini, Statuti... op.cit., p. 93 r, v.

9. "pazzo", verrückt, stammt vom lateinischen "patiens", leidend.

10. "...wie es häufig geschieht, daß durch die Gnade Gottes, unseres Herrn, mit dem Mittel der guten Führung und der Sorgfalt, die man hier anwendet, viele genesen und zu ihren Tätigkeiten zurückkehren." Ordini, Statuti... op. cit., p. 93v. Auch hier steht die soziale Perspektive, daß viele Irre "zu ihren Tätigkeiten zurückkehren" können, im Vordergrund.

11. Es handelt sich um 6 Bände, die Dekrete, Mandate, Inventar usw. registrieren, sowie um 9 Bücher über die Buchhaltung.

12. Libro di decreti del hospitale de S. Maria della Pietà et poveri forestieri et pazzi. 1569-1578, Blatt 124/125. Die Zahlen beziehen sich auf die Gesamtzahl der Hospitalinsassen, die unter dem Titel "pazzi" zusammengefaßt sind.

13. Die Zahlen sind im ersten und dritten der von Ruggiero Pastura veröffentlichten Texte aufgeführt (siehe Anm. 14).

14. Diese Manuskripte wurden zufällig anläßlich der Neuordnung des Barnabiter Archivs aufgefunden und 1972 von Frau Ruggiero Pastura veröffentlicht. Nach ihren Vermutungen und Recherchen handelt es sich beim zweiten und dritten Text um von einem Notar aufgesetzte Schriftstücke. Beide beziehen sich auf eine Visite im Hospital. Der zweite Text ist datiert vom 12.3.1592, er schildert den Zustand und das Inventar der zugehörigen Kirche. Beim dritten Text handelt es sich um eine Bilanz über Ausgaben und Einnahmen des Hospitals. Der vierte Text ist von anderer Hand geschrieben, weder signiert noch datiert, bezieht sich aber inhaltlich auf die gleiche apostolische Visite und auf die erst kurze Amtszeit des neuen Papstes, Clemens VIII. Er dürfte kurz nach den beiden andern Texten geschrieben worden sein. Auch der erste Text ist unsigniert und läßt sich chronologisch nicht eeinordnen, steht aber inhaltich mit den andern Texten in engem Zusammenhang. Für uns von Bedeutung sind vor allem der erste und der vierte Text, die direkt Bezug nehmen auf die Situation im Hospital. Ruggiero Pastura, M.G.: Una "visita" del 1592 all'ospedale dei "Pazzarelli" di Roma, Rassegna degli Archivi di Stato, 1, 1972, p. 46-67.

15. op.cit., p. 61.

16. In einem nicht datierten Brief, der etwa aus der Zeit um 1592 stammen muß, fragen die Bediensteten von S. Maria

della Pietà bei den apostolischen Visitatoren an, ob sie auch mit Zwangmaßnahmen von den Verwandten eines im Hospital untergebrachten Giacomo Toscanella die Pension für ihn und für seinen Diener (!) eintreiben dürften. Brief adressiert: "All Ill.mo et R.mo Sig.ne (Name fehlt)", ASR; Congregazione dell'oratorio; S. Maria in Vallicella, filza 140, c. 85.

Auch wird im Text 4 bei Ruggiero Pastura die Tatsache erwähnt, daß viele Verrückte monatliche Unterhaltszahlungen leisten, op. cit., p. 67.

17. Regole et Ordini, Per il buon governo della Chiesa, & Ospitale della Santissima Pietà, dove si governano, e mantengono gli Huomini, e Donne Pazze della Città di Roma in Piazza Colonna, stabilite al primo d'Ottobre 1635. D'Ordine dell'Eminentissimo Sig. Card. Francesco Barberini, Rom 1635. ASV, Arm. IV, t.9, p.102-112v.

18. Alle Zitate: op. cit., p.110r.

19. Das geht hervor aus einem Bericht der apostolischen Visite von 1630, wo von 43 namentlich genannten Männern 15 aufgezählt werden , die gänzlich auf Kosten des Hospitals leben, genauso wie 14 von den 22 hospitalisierten Frauen. Visitatio Ecclesiae & Domus Hospitalis Stae Mariae Pietatis Dementium, Die 22 Novembris 1630. ASV, Arm. VII, t.113, p. 241-244v.
20. Regole et Ordini... op.cit., p. 106r.

21. Gleichzeitig wird in den "somatischen" Spitälern Roms großer Wert darauf gelegt, daß Ärzte über Aufnahme und allfällige Triage in das zuständige spezialisierte Krankenhaus entscheiden.

22. Regole et Ordini... op. cit., p. 106 r.

23. op. cit., p. 106r,v.

24. "Frauen sind in einem völlig abgetrennten und geschlossenen Teil des Hospitals unterzubringen, der nur

durch eine Tür zugänglich ist und der keine Fenster zum Männerhospital hat. Die Frauen stehen unter der Fürsorge und Wache der Priora, die den Hausschlüssel hat... Wenn die Zahl der Frauen unvertretbar groß wird, kann ihr (der Priora) eine Helferin zur Seite gestellt werden, was gewöhnlich aber nicht für nötig erachtet wird, weil in der Regel die Zahl der verrückten Frauen klein ist und weil sie auch mehr auf blöde Art verrückt werden denn als Rasende. Deshalb kann man die besagten verrückten Frauen zu verschiedenen nötigen Leistungen im Haus einsetzen ohne die Ausgaben des Hospitals zu vergrößern." (!) op.cit., p. 107v, 108r.

25. op.cit., 110v, 111r.

26. Die Abkehr von einer Charakteristik durch materielle Armut zeigt sich sehr schön im Traktat von Fanucci, der 1601 die Irren durch Armut an Hirn definiert: "tutti quelli que sono poveri di cervello". Fanucci, C.: Trattato di tutte le opere pie dell'alma città di Roma, Rom 1601.

27. Die folgenden Ausführungen stützen sich in erster Linie auf folgende Literatur: Comune di Roma: Regesti di Bandi, Editti, Notificazioni e provvedimenti diversi, Rom 1926. Delumeau, J.: Vie économique et sociale de Rome dans la seconde moitié du XVIe siècle, I und II, Paris 1957. Geremek, B.: Il pauperismo nella età preindustriale. In: Storia d'Italia V, Torino 1973, p.669-698. Ginzburg, C.: L'alto e il basso, Aut Aut 181, 1981, p. 3-17. Köhler, E.: Arme und Irre, Berlin 1977. Mollat, M.: I Poveri nel Medioevo, Bari 1982. Petrocchi, M.: Roma nel Seicento, Bologna 1975. Piazza, C.: Eusevologio romano, Rom 1693. Pullan, B.: The old catholiscism, the new catholicism, and the poor. In: Timore e carità. Cremona 1982. Ricci, G.: Povertà, vergogna e povertà vergognosa, Società e storia 5, 1979, p. 305-337.

28. Delumeau berechnet, daß allein im Zeitraum vom 17.1.1582 bis zum 17.1.1583 5942 Personen wegen Schulden inhaftiert waren. Das sind sechs Prozent der damaligen Stadtbevölkerung. Delumeau, op.cit.,p. 498.

29. Simoncelli, P.: Note sul sistema assistenziale a Roma nel XVI secolo. In: Timore e carità, Cremona 1982, p. 137-156, p.144.

30. Simoncelli, P.: Origini e primi anni di vita dell'Ospedale romano dei poveri mendicanti. In: Annuario dell'Istituto storico italiano per l'età moderna e contemporanea, Rom 1976, p. 121-172.

31. Simoncelli, P.: Note... op.cit., p. 155.

32. Rosa, M.: Chiesa, idee sui poveri e assistenza in Italia dal cinque al settecento, Società e storia, 10, 1980, p. 775-806, p.796.

32. Die Polemik geht nicht nur darum, daß die Armen keine Leistung erbringen - arbeitsscheu und faul sind, wie der Vorwurf immer wieder lautet -, sondern auch darum, daß sie nicht die richtige Leistung erbringen. Arbeit als Bettler, Diebe, Simulanten führt gerade zur Attribuierung der falschen Armut. Im Zentrum steht nicht die Besorgnis, daß alle - z. B. auch, indem sie Krankheiten vortäuschend das Mitleid anderer erregen - überleben können, im Zentrum steht das klare Ziel, die Armen zu frommen und demütigen, mit ihrer Armut zufriedenen und arbeitsamen Wesen zu machen. Dazu muß ihre Freiheit gebrochen werden, sich selbständig eine Überleensstrategie aufzubauen. Die Freiheit der Armen ist gleichbedeutend mit der Gefahr moralischer und politischer Unordnung. Die Armen sind gefährlich geworden, deshalb müssen sie eingesperrt und diszipliniert werden.

Kardinal Bellarmino von den Jesuiten ist sich durchaus klar über das Programm, wenn er 1602 festlegt: "Die Armen müssen leben wie Arme, sie müssen sich ihrem Stand entsprechend kleiden und so spielen, wie es ihrem Stand entspricht. Viele werden daher Bettler und ruinieren ihre Sachen, weil sie mehr ausgeben wollen, als ihnen zusteht: fürs Essen, für die Kleidung, fürs Spielen und für die Mitgift Ihrer Töchter. Wenn sie sich mit ihrem Status zufrieden gäben, würde Gott ihnen mehr helfen, als er es jetzt tut." R. Bellarmino, Opera oratoria V.Zit. nach: Fioriani, L.: Religione e povertà. Ricerche per la storia religiosa di Roma 3, Rom 1979, p. 59.

Erweiter Text und ausführliches Literaturverzeichnis beim Verfasser.

The Concept of Madness and its Implications in Talmudic Literature and Exegeses

M. Ganek

Summary: In spite of their spatial and temporal dispersion, the Talmudic literature and its commentaries proceed from a fundamental unity.

On one hand, the definitions of madness are, a priori, extremely rigid; originally, they were exemplars, quoted to resolve practical problems.

On the other hand, the handling of these definitions requires a very important suppleness in the jurisprudence of legal implications of madness. Obviously, the dialectics of the rabbi's show the care to respect the personal life of the individual and the spiritual life of the community.

And if these conceptions have still an application nowadays, that is because the Talmud speaks of the mad and not of the mental ill without any cross-checking between the socio-legal model of madness and the medical model.

WE WOULD LIKE TO TRY and give an outline of the concept of madness in Talmudic literature and its exegeses.

These exegeses have been drawn up over a period of practically two thousand years, up to our epoch, and their authors resided all around the world; but although coming from societies temporally and spatially very far apart, this literature testifies, however, to a fundamental and indisputable unity.

All this literature in effect is supported by the Talmud - this literary monument of Palestinian and Babylonian rabbis at the dawn of Christian era - written to make, of one part, the sum of all the oral laws not yet drawn up, but that could sometimes be so ancient that we considered them as being delivered to Moses by God on Mount Sinai; on the other part, to become complete and to explain certain passages of the delicate interpretation of the Bible and of the Michna. The Talmud thus, in a way, represents the Humanities of the Jewish people, an Encyclopedia, series of essentially theological preoccupations, but it also treats all sectors of spiritual life and of practical life. And it is thanks to the Talmud that the Jewish people, deprived of national ground, would find the cultural cement explaining its remarkable power of cohesion and resistance, all the long of the Diaspora.

In effect, at all times in all countries, the trustees of the law, the guides of the Jewish people, with the knowledge of the rabbis, would, in the light of the Bible and the Talmud, find the base for their decisions. Indeed, the evolution of customs and civilization would pose new problems, but essentially, these problems were elucidated, not by the light of contemporary acquisitions, that were philosophical or even scientific, but always in the light of the writings themselves, in respecting the original spirit of these, and, for as much as it was possible, the same letter. The rabbinical Responsa thus searches, in difficult cases, for an interpretation of an ancient text, to adopt to a new situation created by the evolution of civilization.

Our study thus embraces all the traditional Jewish literature, since the Bible, up to certain rabbinical Responsa written eventually in our days; but we don't understand the practice of a historic division, that was purely artificial and often betrays the spirit of these texts inspired by the same source.

Likewise, it is evident that, by the traditional Jewish literature, we exclusively understand Biblical and Talmudic literature, or issues like this and we don't allow for scientific or medical works, eventually written by a theologian of the Jewish tradition, but founded on science or medicine in the vigor of the era of its editor.

However, this traditional literature does not behave as the treaty of medicine, even less than psychiatry. The problem of madness is accosted in relation with practical cases, as such that the legal validity of acts committed by mad people, such as the care or the attention that demands it, an ethical, and not medical, point of view. This problem does not inscribe, not in a therapeutic context, nor to even properly speak in a diagnostic context.

The Talmud is a legal work, founded on theology, and the bearing of the legislature is absolutely not that of the psychiatrist; we could qualify it in the opposite way. For the psychiatrist, the definition of madness is advanced and sensitive; it is in fact by a precocious and appropriate diagnostic formulation that the therapeutic chances are increased.

But for the wise Talmudist, if he declares an individual mad, its only after defining what legal, social, and religious acts would be invalidated by his state; after defining the duties which society has freed for his regard, or on the contrary the new duties that devolved upon it. In this precise context, it is not a question of finesse or of precociousness in the diagnosis. So much as a subject understands the legal or religious range of the act he commits, he is not considered as mad - or legal invalid - at least opposite of this act, even if his behavior and his understanding, excludes all participation in public life. The good Talmudist looks to recoil the limits of madness, in that which concerns its socio-legal meaning.

The critical and reflective bearings of the Talmudist is absolutely not that of a semiological analysis. Practically, the problem posed is this: being given an individual who is considered mad by society, according to which criteria will they judge his madness? It thus acts as a subject presenting a spectacular and massive pathology, where they document characteristics and pathognomic signs of his madness.

But this resolution of madness in one or some pathognomic signs, does not teach us about madness for its own sake, and for another thing, leads to risk of abuse. In effect, in our day, it is the doctor who decides, by a medical process, if there is or is not mental illness, eventually interlocking with a legal process, the wise Talmudists, be they doctors or not, have to decide, not only the legal consequences of madness, but madness itself. They thus employ, in minute analysis the base criteria, to limit as much of the abuse as possible.

Finally, the way of editing both the Talmud and the rabbinical Responsa is the source of new hazards: The Talmud, in effect, was not written by a systematic codification, but following an collaborative method and under the form of dialogues. We slide from one subject to another, by citing the opinion of someone else. The rabbis, in their Responsa, generally consider individual questioners, and without the general rules given for an impersonal application.

The problems posed are resolved by always referring to the legal precedents, thus the analogy is sometimes simply formal.

Even more, the context of the considered case is rarely mentioned; now, the context is essential, because it's he who, as a last resort, poses the problem. And we can legitimately suppose that a more or less compensated neurosis, or more exactly a compensated neurotic subject, has never been made the object of legislation.

After all the necessary preliminaries, it becomes evident that we are not searching for a "translation", in psychiatric symptoms or syndromes, the descriptions, often in very clear view, made by the Talmud, except in passing, when the context precisely permits it. We search to prove the critical and reflective bearings that the wise Jews confronted with the definitions that finally represent the extreme boundaries of madness and its stumbling block.

Finally, with the concerns of clarity, we are permitted to successively study the criterias of madness, for the social, legal and religious consequences of the status of madness, although in traditional literature these problems are always inseparable. But the complexity of the considered cases it that of a clear comprehension necessarily passed by this dichotomy.

Criteria of Madness

1) At the base of all the discussion arising around madness, is a fundamental definition, extremely succinct.

"What is a mad person? He that goes out only at night, he who sleeps in cemeteries, he who rips his clothing." (Talmud of Babylon, Hagiga 3b 4a)

It is probable that these three behaviors represent only examples at the moment of the editing of the Talmud; it must in addition, to appreciate them for their proper value, know that they denote a great oddness. But above all, as we will see, these behaviors do not sum up madness; these are not medical models. They are delivered to us, on the contrary, as a limited frontier of madness. The Talmud pursues:

> It was taught as follows: Rav Houna (1) says the three signs must be combined. Rabbi Yohanan (2) declared: 'Just one of these signs is sufficient.'
>
> How does the case present itself in practice?
>
> - for one thing, if he acts like a mad person, just one of these acts would be significant;

- but on the other hand, if he committed these three acts in a normal manner, the combination of the three, in this case would be significant.

To tell the truth, it acts in someone who does these acts in a mad manner, for:

- if he sleeps in cemeteries, we could claim a 'grandipass' (an illness provoked by a strong agony) had seized him;
- if he tears his clothes, we could object he is absorbed in his thoughts;
- but if he commits these three acts, he is considered as the ox who gores an ox, a donkey and a camel and he is thus plainly responsible.

Two general lines of contrary interpretation appear, in the function of the context; but above all, he must have a spirit which does not act in a medical description and argumentation, but the legal base of jurisdictions; and its thus that Rachi (3) - who in his criticisms of the Talmud of Babylon cites the difficult passages and explains them - precisely from the outset:

> What is a mad person? This question is mentioned everywhere after exempting the religious commandments and punishments (to violate the commandments) the subject recognizes madness, and after all the acts of acquisition or sale effected by him are void.

Anyhow, we must not see in these behaviors an indelible seal of madness, and the editors, then the commentators, clearly stating these behaviors well, taken one by one, can justify it. It becomes highly probable that if someone committed these three acts he would thus be acting as a mad person.

"As for the reference - the legal value - to the ox goring the ox, donkey and camel", it provides the formal similarity between the two cases: according to biblical legislation, a goring ox must not be fundamentally held for goring until the third offense, and the law distinguishes between the goring ox in comparison to one or all species of animals.

This formal similarity is of the origin of a putting into parallel even more pushed in the Tossefot (4):

> If he does these acts like a mad person, just one of these acts is significant; but the following question is posed:
>
> - must they obtain the definitive status of madness, uniquely as to this act, being given that it takes three different acts to consider them as mad in general, in the same way as the goring isn't in plain

responsibility in comparison to all the species of animals as he gores the ox, donkey and camel.

It is evident that this discussion is absolutely not of the medical order; it has no sense. But it acts, for the Tossefot, to appreciate if this type of madness must exclude the subject from all community life, or simply from a certain category of acts in relation with their type of madness. The Tossefot, searching to guaranteed spiritual integrity of the accomplishment of a religious or legal act, prefers to consider the subject not as "partially mad", but as "mad in comparison to all items" ; but the Tossefot states well "just one act committed one time is not sufficient to give him the definitive status of madness."

In fact, to decide this, the Tossefot obviously leans on the Talmud; after the discussion between Rav Houna and Rabbi Yohanan, the Talmud continues after all:

Rav Papa (5) says: 'if only Rav Houna had heard what was taught in a Beraita: - what is a mad person? He who loses that which he is given' -, he would take back the opinion he had given.

Otherwise said, there exists an anterior text - and which, because it is anterior, has the power of law - deciding madness in a unique category of acts; and those of the Tossefot, by the same reasoning, concluded that just one of these behaviors of the basic definition suffices to affirm a subject is mad in a general manner.

Thus we see in Talmudic literature discussions at length of the value to grant a certain act in accordance to how it was committed, according to the context, according to the repetition. This appears, indeed, at first look as a sterile edict, and in all cases without psychiatric interest. But, once again, it is not in therapy that the wise Talmudists exist; they are in depositories of the law and, as such, must be respected. But this respect for the law does not serve but to hurt the rights of the individual. This explains the minute almost obsessional arguments, induced by the terse brevity is itself necessary, for it is this that permits the legislators to liberally judge each case, all in referring to the legitimacy of a basic text.

We can ask of what value the reference has to a model of madness drawn up in the 2nd century A.D., and to what standards should all the decision makers arrive at, be it their century, be it their country of adoption.

The Talmud of Jerusalem, contemporary of the Talmud of Babylon, equally studies the definition of madness on these same bases, but introduces different developments. The Talmud of Jerusalem proposes, in regard to the base behaviors:

> Rav Houna said: It must be the meeting of all the signs, if not I could pretend that:
> - he who goes out at night is a 'kynitrokos,'
> - he who sleeps in cemeteries sacrifices to the demons,
> - he who tears his clothing is 'solikos,'
> - he who loses all he is given is 'codeicos'.

It is difficult to know to what these terms correspond to, probably derived from Greek and several times distorted: The commentator Pne Moche (6) states:

> Kynitrokos: other version of controkos, other version of canitrophos (corresponding to the grandipass of the Talmud of Babylon.)
>
> Solikos: other version of colikos, kinokos.
>
> Codeicos or cordeicos: other version of cobicos, playing with dice and losing all his money.

If the first term has an indisputable relation with cynicism, and if the sense of the last term is known, the etymology finally matters little; the essence is that, for the Talmud of Jerusalem, the cordeicos represents, as we will see, a form of mental illness, that for as much as it does not grant to that which is reaches the legal state of madness. This is a fundamental demarcation between the clinical sense of mental illness and the legal sense of madness.

In effect, the Talmud of Jerusalem continues:

> However the cordeicos presents none of these symptoms.
>
> But what is a cordeicos?
>
> Rabbi Yossi says 'Hamim' (dull, confused, petrified)
>
> A case was presented before Rabbi Yossi: a resident of the Tarse, to whom we gave the red in the black, and he remained confused, of black in the red, and he remained confused; Rabbi Yossi says: It's the cordeicos of whom the good speak.

The number of commentators, in following this, searched to further state what was the cordeicos; for Rochi, it acts as a demon - a term not to be taken by the letter, but understood as a mental derangement, - which seized he who drank lots of wine freshly drawn from the vat.

For Maimonide (8): "Illness that comes from a fullness of cerebral ventricles, troubles the spirit and provokes a crisis of epilepsy."

If the sages do not fall exactly in agreement with the nature of the illness as represented in the cordeicos, it is indisputable that it is a result of mental pathology, a notion already evident in the Talmud of Babylon, which expresses it in this manner:

> Rech Lakich (9) says that the cordeïcos is similar to a man who sleeps.
>
> Rabbi Yohanan says the cordeicos is similar to madness.
>
> Why does Rabbi Yohanan not consider it as a man who sleeps? For a man who sleeps has no need for treatment to recover his full conscience, and the cordeicos has need for treatment.
>
> Why does Rech Lakich not consider it as madness? For the mad person, we do not possess a treatment to heal them; but for this one, the medication is in our hands.

We must know that this discussion makes implicit reference to the legislation on divorce; or as we will see later, we cannot allow a divorce to the wife of a mad person; but on the other hand, we can allow a divorce to a woman, with the consent of her husband, even when he is asleep. Comparing the cordeicos with the man who sleeps, Rech Lakich thus does not consider him as mad.

The gaps between the preoccupations of the Talmudist, the legislators, and those of the doctor are thus very clear. All of these authors admit that the cordeicos indisputably presents a mental pathology; but it is not "sufficiently mad" in this way, to be liable to an expulsion looking to deprive him of a certain number of his rights. The fact that the cordeicos is assuredly curable forces us to not consider him as mad.

If the succinct character of the fundamental definitions originates through an extremely circumstantiated interpretation, it is, however, arrived at by a sage presented as a double polarity of preoccupations, legal and medical. This is the case of Maimonide, who, being a great legislator of Judaism, is also a doctor of great reputation, and finds himself many times opposed to other legislators due to the interpretation given to Talmudic definitions.

In Beit -Yossef (10), we indeed read:

> According to Maimonide, the signs mentioned in the Hagiga treaty, the leaving at night, the losing of objects, the sleeping in cemeteries, the ripping of clothes, are all only examples and it is the same for all acts of madness. But according to Rabenou Simha (11) and Rabenou Avigdor Cohen (12), cited by Rav I. Kolon (13), principal 19, in relation to an act of divorce given to Witzbourg, if his madness is not characterized by the signs mentioned in the Hagiga treaty, he must be considered as normal.

It is clear that for Maimonide, doctor, these signs do not summarize madness; but Maimonide, legislator, is held to refer to madness from the Talmud decrees on madness. And although, in the text cited, Maimonide speaks before all as long as is legislated, the fact that the Talmud is a subject for which many interpretations are permitted, with the condition of respecting the internal coherence of the Talmud, to give an interpretation that remains legitimate and is equally satisfying in the eyes of a doctor. Contrary to this, Rabenou Simha and Rav Avigdor Cohen, only being legislators, cannot permit themselves to get past the strict frame of Talmudic examples, which, for them, dwells in the codification of laws.

Evidently, the opinion of Maimonide is much more satisfying on the scientific plane; and it is the occasion to remember that Maimonide probably returns here to the spirit of the editors of the Talmud, for who these behaviours certainly only represent examples. Always it is the opinion of Maimonide that is generally accepted, and more and more, what he does at the actual hour, where his texts are long from being dead letters, a satisfying interpretation for the modern spirit is totally legitimate.

2) Two other categories of subjects generally are liable to the same laws of madness, and forms with it, in the Talmudic legislation, a triptych. They are the child and the deaf and dumb. We must not hastily deduce that the Talmud sees the child and the deaf and dumb as mad people. Much more simply, the child is considered as a legal invalid, awaiting his intellectual development and his maturity.

The problem is more difficult for the deaf and dumb; on one side, the same Hebrew term Heresh is used in Talmudic literature to generally designate the deaf and dumb, but sometimes only the deaf; on the other hand, the context sometimes makes proof that this same term is employed to designate the dumb. In these two cases, the approach is not medical, but social-legal.

For he who is isolated by being dumb, without being deaf the Talmud considers above all the subjects brutally beaten, and the legislator looks to mark the limits of what designates being dumb; otherwise said, is it a cerebral or mental attack? In effect the sages suspect a process that could bring together an organic or an hysterical aphasia, seen apart from autism. And thus they imagined the tests after judging the intellectual faculties of the subject, knowing by experience the cases of total healing, without aftermath, in the case of being dumb. As always, it acts in fact from an essentially practical problem posed at the origin by a dumb person wishing to agree to a divorce from his wife (Michna Gittin 7,1).

> A man is stricken with being dumb. We ask him
>
> - Do you wish us to write the act of divorce for your wife?
>
> If he nods his head affirmative, we ask him three different questions; if he answers no when he should, and yes when he should, we can draw up the act of divorce and pronounce it.

For more security, Rachi gives three questions with a positive response and three with a negative one; the Talmud itself considers the test indicated by Michna as insufficient (Talmud of Babylon, Gittin 70 b):

> Maybe he has an 'inclination of the head' towards yes, or the reverse, no?

(The term we translated by inclination is, according to Rachi, a mental illness to always reply yes with the head, to whatever question it may be, or always no, and its relation with the content of the question.) To prevent a certain case the Talmud thus imposes a more complex rhythm of answers, that the Tossefot would take back and would further elaborate for even more security.

Finally, the problem of the dumb person is quite simple and coherent; if being dumb inscribes in the more vast frame a cerebral or mental attack, the subject effectively brings together madness, in all cases in that which concerns the jurisdiction to which he is submitted; on the other hand, if the subject makes proof, to the aid of the proposed tests, of an isolated dumb person, without any intellectual problem, the jurisdiction on which he depends would be clearly different than that of a mad person.

In that which concerns the deaf and dumb, it is evident that someone deaf and dumb from birth could involve a slow intellectual development bordering on mental backwardness, effectively approaching the subject of madness. In a more general manner, the deaf and dumb person would be excluded from the tasks done in the name of the community, but having however, in that which concerns his personal life, a certain number of prerogatives that the mad person does not have.

3) The reflective bearing of the sage Talmudists appears thus animated by two principal directors, who conduct them to surround themselves with a maximum of precautions before eventually pronouncing the exclusion of a subject; to one end it finds the worry of defending the authenticity of the religious and social life of the community, thus explaining the prohibitions made to the mad person, to the dumb and deaf and to the child acting in the name of this. To the other pole there is the worry of defending the humane person, thus explaining the tendency of sages to clearly make the distinction between the mad person and the deaf and dumb person, and above all to push back as much as possible the legal limits of madness.

This permissivity in respect of the mad person remarkably illustrated in the instructive text in respect of King Solomon, and which indisputably evokes for the psychiatrist a systematic frenzy, or maybe a fantastic frenzy.

The Talmud in effect reports that King Solomon was dispossessed from his throne by an impostor, and he was poorly clothed, in the country, in invariably defending the fact that he was the king. We do not consider him invariably as a mad person. Now history reaches to Sanhedrin - the supreme institution of the Sages - who, were well informed "A mad person does not attach himself to a only one topic", wondered who could be the claimant on the throne, surveyed the impostor, and finally demasked him.

Rachi estimates, on this subject, that someone whose behavior is usually quite normal, and who attaches himself to saying a lone and sole inept action, during his life, cannot be mad.

This legend indeed does not have the force of law, the opinion of Rachi is perhaps disputable in the matters of psychiatry, but this legend is representative of the spirit in which the sages look to comprehend madness.

In effect, the paranoid worries can, through its coherence and interior logic, be imposing on the observer; or again in fantastic frenzy, that which strikes, is the contrast seizing between the paralogical conceptions and the mythology of frenzy, and a correct (and sometimes perfect) adaptation to the real. Now, for the legislator, the important part is precisely this adaptation to the real, or at least the coherence and the logic of reasoning, which permits to affirm that in a different field of the conscience - in the occurrence of religious practice -, there is no interference between the eventual frenzy and the accomplishment of religious acts. That he is frenzied, so be it, but the important thing is that this frenzy leaves the subject to normally accomplish his duties, in having conscience of what he does, and there is no doubt that in that which concerns his social and religious insertion the subject would not be regarded as mad by the wise Talmudist.

4) It is always this double individual - society polarity that brings the sages to study periodic madness, in the more general sense and in the more vague of terms. He does not need to know more if the subject is mad, but when he is mad, otherwise said, it is the legal validity of his acts in the function of the evolution of his state.

There, more again than before, we enter the domain of the practical applications of the legislation, encroaching in fact on the implications of madness that we will see afterwards. But we have believed it good to place here a few of the cases after stressing the critical and reflective bearing of the Talmudists.

In the Talmud of Babylon, it is a question of the man who, at the time of an epileptic crisis, ate some Matsa (azyme bread). By doing this does he accomplish his religious obligation, or does he have to eat it again once more once he has recovered his lucidity?

> He was taught: he who is sometimes well taken, sometimes mad, is considered as lucid as to all these acts when he is well taken, and when he is mad, is considered as mad as to all these acts.

In regard to the sale of goods:

> A man inclined to madness sold his goods; if the testimony attests that this sale was affected by a state of madness, it is invalidated. (Talmud of Babylon)

Or again, in regard to divorce (14):

When a man is in a period of lucidity, he can grant the divorce. And it suffices for this that he is, for the most part, well taken. If he is not completely lucid, it is not necessary to give him examinations as one would with a dumb person; he is considered well taken if he behaves normally, without tearing his clothes, without going to the cemetery, etc... and this, even if he is weakened, if the signs of the illness persist, if he is not completely cured, with the condition that he is already in a phase of convalescence, he is considered as well taken.

It is there again that the reference to Talmudic criteria permits Rachba to not consider the subject as mad, even though clinically some doubts towards his state persist.

Finally Maimonide, in the laws of the testimonies, says:

The epileptic during a crisis is invalid to testify, but as soon as he is recovered he is suitable to testify, and that which acts of a subject having crises periodically or not. This, to the condition that his spirit is not constantly troubled, for there exist epileptics whose spirit is troubled even outside of a crisis. And it suits to consider with much circumspection all testimonies of the epileptic.

Once again, strong in his medical knowledge, Maimonide isolates little of the Talmud - all in respecting its legitimacy - to permit an appreciation more fully of the epileptics circumstances.

Social, Legal and Religious Implications of Madness

1) Sale or acquisition of goods

We have seen that all sales or acquisitions of goods effectuated by a mad person are legally void.

2) Therapeutic responsibilities towards a mad person

The preoccupations of the Talmud in regard to the mad person remarkably illustrate in regard to their therapeutic preoccupations; once again, it is an ethical problem that is raised and not a medical problem; the Talmud absolutely does not search to define which treatment to apply, but by whom care and attention should be provided to the mad person.

The problem is clearly stated in the Talmud of Babylon, under the form of an anecdote, but this anecdote is fundamental for in fact it represents the legal precedent.

> Rav Assi (15) had an old mother. She said to him 'I want jewels.' He gave them to her. She said to him 'I want you to find me a husband' and he said 'We will look for one for you.' She said 'I want him to be as handsome as you.' He abandoned her and rose in Israel.

The reaction of Rav Assi is 'a priori' totally surprising, but the comments explain very clearly; thus, in the Tossefot, Rabbi Itshak of the ancient remarks:

> When she desired a man as handsome as him, to this he recognized her spirit was troubled and he ran away, seeing he could not accomplish his obligations to the regard of the sky.

Otherwise said, for Rabbi Itshak of antiquity (16), Rav Assi would inevitably, one day or another, be compelled to violate the divine commandment to respect ones' parents, that which amply justified his leaving.

Maimonide is more precise:

> He whose father or mother has a troubled spirit must try hard to conduct themselves to their regard according to their desires up until they are taken in mercy. If it is impossible to hold this bet because their spirit is too troubled, that he abandons them and orders others to occupy themselves with them as he would do.

However, for Rabbi Avraham Ben David, of Posquieres (17), if the attitude of Rav Assi is justified by particular circumstances, this is not a sufficient reason to make a general guide, and he objects to Maimonide:

> This is not a guide of value; if he abandons them, who can he command to look after them?

For him, it is evident that if the son of a mad person is unable to occupy himself with them, no one would accept to do it.

This argument is refuted by Rabbi David Ben Zimra (18), who confirms the opinion of Maimonide:

> I don't know why Rabbi Avraham Ben David says that its an incorrect law and assuredly, that which Rav Assi does, to order others to occupy themselves by means of salary, is justified. And this was for his good, for, with regard to his son, he was full of tenderness and had not shame for him, that which is not the case towards others; on the other hand, his son could not scold, so that others could shout, and even punishment by blows, that which would bring healing, cases that we run into often enough, so that the son could absolutely not act in this way.

Two theses thus are confronted, one praising the responsibility and direct commitment of the son, the other praising competence and efficiency.

One more time, the direct drawing up one of the anecdote of Rav Assi recovers a fundamental ethical problem, that is not presented by the great analogy with the case, in our days, of a doctor, treating or not treating his own family.

3) The compensation for damage from madness.

After the Hebrew legislation, he who brings bodily harm unto another is held legally to shed repairs for:

- care made necessary by the damage done,
- temporary incapacity to work
- the pretium doloris
- permanent bodily invalidity
- and finally the "price of shame"

The Talmud states:

> He who shames a mad person is dispensed to pay the compensation.

That is to say, he who is responsible for physical damage done by a mad person would only be held to shed the first four indemnities. The Talmud makes the distinction between the subjective sentiment of shame, and the objective sentiment, defined by the norms of society, as much as the subject can keep from taking it to heart. For the Talmud, "a mad person cannot be hurt in his honor", "for there is no greater shame than to be mad", and he thus does not compensate him, even if he feels the subjective sentiment.

The Michna equally states:

> A hitch with the deaf and dumb person, the mad person, the child, is unlucky for, he who hurts them, must compensate them, for they are exempt.

4) Marriage

From the Tora, the deaf and dumb are like mad people and cannot contract marriage. However, by rabbinical institution, the sages brought an amendment in that which concerns deaf and dumb people and validated their marriage.

> Why do the sages not institute a marriage between mad people, the same as for deaf and dumb people? It is the rabbinical institution of madness of these that is practical, and that's why the sages created for them the possibility of marrying. It is not the same for mad people who do not respect rabbinical institutions.

It is not eugenic considerations which here guide the sages, but humanitarian considerations; the Talmud, estimating that we "are not alive with a serpent on our roof", presumes that a couple with one mad person would not be discordant. And Rachi, in his criticisms, stresses there is no reason to think that a couple in which one is mad, would not behave in harmony, when this harmony is not menaced by deafness and dumbness of one or the other spouse.

It is different in that which concerns epileptics:

> A man would not marry a woman belonging to a family of epileptics. This is affirmed when the case is presented three times.

And Rabbi Yossef Caro states that, by there, he must hear the three times it is repeated in the case of children born of this union, themselves epileptic.

5) Divorce

Divorce, complex in itself, becomes extremely complex in relation with madness. It does not have the symmetry between man and woman in the traditional Jewish legislation; divorce is always and necessarily a voluntary act on the part of the man, as the woman can be repudiated.

We have already seen that if a dumb person - and this is equally true of the deaf and dumb person - can make proof of the integrity of his intellectual faculties the divorce can be granted.

In return, for the cordeicos:

> If a man stricken with a cordeicos gives the order to write an act of divorce for his wife, the act is without value.
>
> If someone gives the order to write an act of divorce for his wife, and is then taken by a cordeicos, and he says 'do not draw up this act' this last subject is without value.

Maimonide, in addition, generalizes the problem of cordeicos in the form of transitory mental derangement.

Finally, the divorce in the case of the husband being mad is very simple: for the divorced to be recognized as being legitimate, it must be certain that we know the decision was made in full knowledge of the cause, and the sages look to protect the spiritual authenticity of the divorce.

For the woman, the reflective bearing is very different; The Talmud looks to protect the individual, with the knowledge of the mad woman, who, repudiated, would be without defense in life.

We have seen that a mad person cannot contract a marriage; but the Talmud states:

> If he is married to a lucid woman who afterwards becomes mad, he is forbidden to divorce her. According to the Tora, he is permitted to divorce her in a similar case, but this is a rabbinical institution, so that people do not abuse her.

It acts there again as a rabbinical amendment dedicated to protect the woman. The decision makers wanted to avoid placing the woman in the margin of society; but on the other hand, conscious of the burden this would present for the husband, they state the legislation referring to the conditions of divorce such as were stated in the Tora; thus, according to the Tora, divorce is ratified by two clauses:

- by the gift of the document of divorce to the woman, if this is capable of receiving and keeping the act.

- by the fact that the woman, having received the act of divorce, is in the measure of being sent back and not returning to the primitive focus.

These two clauses, in relation with madness, are considered as two criteria of non-madness, or at least 'a minimal madness, and schematically, three cases are presented:

- the woman is repudiated and incapable of keeping the act, indisputable pledge of madness, and the divorce cannot be pronounced;

- even with mental illness, she is capable to subscribe to the two clauses, and the rabbinical institution thus does not hold, legally, for madness, permitting the pronouncing of the divorce.

- the woman keeps the act of divorce, but cannot keep herself. It is there that the rabbinical institution intervenes to prevent such a divorce.

Maimonide states the spirit in which these laws are drawn up:

> He who marries a woman who has become mad must not divorce her before she is cured. This is a rabbinical institution, so that she is not the prey of perverse people that would abuse her, for she does not know how to keep herself... But the husband is not forced to the three principal marital duties: the feeding, the clothing, and sexual enjoyment, for a sensible man does not have the power to live with

> mad people in the same house. And he is not obligated to cure them nor to rescue them.
>
> But if the divorce is pronounced, she is considered as a divorce, and he must leave the house and is not held to attend to her.

The woman thus brings the marriage into a certain minimal lump sum, the "Ketouba", Maimonide thus states that the husband, if he does not have the legal possibility of divorce, becomes in a way the legal guardian of his wife, but is no longer held to provide care for his wife with his own money, nor to pay a ransom if she is a captive; the money of the Ketouba serves to pay all these ends.

It suffices to say that certain decision makers do not agree with Maimonide, and certain points remain controversial:

- that which concerns financial obligations, and some consider they fall due to the husband with his own money.
- for some, the divorce in any case cannot be pronounced.

And finally, the legislation on divorce testifies once again this individual-society double polarity: For the man, the sages search to preserve the authenticity of the act of divorce, that is to say the society; for the woman, it's themselves that the sages protect, precisely against society.

6) The Testimonies

> The mad person is invalid to give testimony, and not only the mad person who walks around naked, but those whose spirit is bewildered, constantly troubled in a certain domain, as much as we can pertinently converse with him in other domains; this one is also considered as mad and is invalid to testify.

As always, doctor Maimonide, all in respecting the internal coherence of the Talmudic legislation, extends the jurisdiction of madness - in the matter of testimonies - to certain subjects who probably don't fall under the domain of strict Talmudic definition. But we have already seen of Maimonide, concerning epileptics in particular, even outside of a crisis, risks to present quite serious troubles, requires an extreme rigor in the choice of witnesses.

However Rabbi Yossef Caro stresses that Maimonide does not pass the frame of Talmudic legality:

> That which our master says, that a lone domain suffices, implies that which acts in the manner of a mad person. Maimonide does not wish to say that a certain act, committed once, makes us consider them as mad, but if this is the custom, as he says himself 'His spirit

> is constantly troubled'; And that which is mentioned in the Talmud, he who loses what he is given... is not specific, but it acts only as examples, that is why our master did not mention them, and was content just to say 'He whose spirit is troubled,' that which equally includes other symptoms.

7) Religion

The reflective bearing of the sages is here and we cannot make it more clear: We must guarantee the spiritual value of the religious act, without hurting the individual. Its thus that:

> All in each is apt to the public lecture of Rouleau d'Esther, except the deaf and dumb, the mad, and the children.

And quite evidently, we cannot give to someone the responsibility of being efficient in the community, if there exists doubt as to whether they understand their own actions.

Exactly with the same logic:

> A deaf and dumb person, a mad person or a child cannot sound the Choraf for the community and to this accomplish his religious duties.

This same logical bearing involves a different attitude in that which concerns ritual slaughter:

> The mad person is unfit to do ritual slaughter, in fear that he would practice it bad. But if others were present at the time of the slaughter, and can attest that it was regular, the slaughter is valid.

Opposite from the two preceding acts, whose value is uniquely spiritual, it is the technique of ritual slaughter, shored up by the knowledge of laws that assume, that is the sponsor for the community and the accomplishment of his duties. The mad person is thus 'a priori' unfit for a certain act, but if, in particular circumstances, he is all the same brought to having practiced, the attestations of the witnesses, as the slaughter is regular, the valid of 'a posterior'.

Finally, in that which concerns the priesthood, the Michna naturally stipulates: "The mad person is unfit to the priesthood". But if a mad person is unfit to the religious vocation, he conserves no less than the hereditary quality of the priest, and thus his privileges are forbidden.

In conclusion we see that the field of application of the definition of madness is necessary to shed light on the critical and reflective bearings of the sages; at no moment do they understand, with the aid of their criteria, the parallels to medicine; their domain is that of the law, and they pose as arbitrators of a limited situation; they never act to precociously detect the first signs of mental illness, but, completely opposite, when the behavior of a subject leaves to assume madness, they must decide if, legally, the subject is mad; they do not act to put the subject at the ban of the community, but to the opposite, all the cases that we have seen show the incessant contact of the mad person and the rest of the community.

It acts to protect the mad person from society against which he cannot defend himself, and it acts to protect society against the degradation of a mad person's spiritual life.

And we conclude that a certain perspective necessitates, more than the text states, more than a minute and definitive labeling of all mad people, a great suppleness in the extemporaneous interpretation of each case and a great opening of the spirit.

The sharp texts define madness in the Talmud responding perfectly to this perspective. Not bothering with a mass of details or with several rigid models of madness, they permit a great suppleness in the manipulation of criteria, and a great latitude of interpretation.

Today these texts are not dead in the Jewish community; indeed they are no longer laws that decide madness, as psychiatrists now do; the legal view does not correspond with the medical diagnosis, and does not eventually count. We should not be astonished: the medical model of mental illness is contrary to views in traditional Jewish literature, which is a socio-legal model of madness.❧

References

1. Rav Houna, 2e génération des Amoraïm, ou sages ayant contribué a la rédaction du Talmud, IIIe siècle, Babylone.

2. Rabbi Yohanan, 2e génération des Amoraïm, IIIe siecle, Palestine.

3. Rachi, Rabbi Salomon Ben Itshak (1040-1105), France, Allemagne; Gloses sur le Talmud de Babylone.

4. Tossefot: Compilation d'auteurs franco-allemands, XIIe-XIIIe siècles.

5. Rav Papa, 5e génération des Amoraïm (?- 386), Palestine.

6. Rabbi Moche Margalit (1710 ou 1720- 1781), Lituhanie, Amsterdam; Pne Moche: commentaire du Talmud de Jerusalem.

7. Rabbi Yossi, 4e génération des Amoraïm, Palestine.

8. Maïmonide (Rabbi Moche Ben Maïmon ou Rambam) (1135- 1203), Espagne, Afrique du Nord, Egypte: Commentaire de la Michna.

9. Rech Lakich: Rabbi Chimon Ben Lakich, 2e génération des Amoraïm, Palestine.

10. Rabbi Yossef Caro (1488-1575), Turquie, Palestine: Beit-Yossef.

11. Rabenou Simha (Rabbi Simha Ben Chemouel, de Vitry) (fin du XIe s., debut XIIe), France.

12. Rabenou Avigdor Cohen (Rav Avigdor Ben Eliahou Cohen), XIIIe s., Autriche.

13. Rav Yossef Kolon (?- 1480), Italie.

14. Rachba (Rabbi Chlomo Ben Abraham Adreth) (1235-1310), Espagne: Responsum 705, Volume 1.

15. Rav Assi, 3e génération des Amoraïm, Palestine.

16. Rabbi Itshak l'Ancien (Rabbi Isaac Ben Samuel, de Dampierre), XIIe s., France.

17. Rabbi Avraham Ben David, de Posquieres (dit Ibn Daud, ou Ravdad) (1120-1198), Posquières, Montpellier.

18. Rabbi David Ben Zimra (1480-1574), Espagne, Palestine.

19. Michna, 1911, Editions Romm, Vilna.

20. Talmud de Babylone, 1895, Editions Romm, Vilna.

21. Talmud de Jérusalem, 1911, Editions Romm, Vilna.

22. Granek M.- Le concept de la folie dans la société juive traditionnelle. Thèse doctorat en médecine, Paris, 1975.

23. Harboun H. - La folie dands la tradition hébraïque. Thèse doctorat en psychopathologie, Sorbonne, 1974.

24. Simon I.- Revue d'histoire de la médecine hébraïque, Paris.

Madness and Witchcraft in the Rio de la Plata in Times of the Inquisition

F. P. Larraya

Summary: We study the Inquisition within the Rio de la Plata area as an exposition of the general dialectic of classicism and mannerism as enunciated by Ernest Robert Curtius, in which madness finds its transcendental meaning. This synthetic essay is based on both archival work, and bibliographical analysis of three invaluable folio books - unknown to date - discovered at the Archdiocese Archives of the Argentine Province of Córdoba.

...After I felt the prison of the stick on my arms and I learned
That my hands without fingers would no longer bleed.
Perhaps I will sleep, perhaps I won't.
I returned from nothing.
I wanted to rebuild the world.

Antonio Di Bendetto

DURING the carnival of 1987, I visited Franca Ongaro, the lady senator for the Sinestra Independent in her mansion in Venice, who worked in the legislative body in the modernization of the "By Law 180", by which asylums were eradicated in Italy.

That visit was to me, like a return to the brief friendship with her husband Franco Basaglia (1924-1980), that was established in a trip from Zürich to Kreuzlingen (1957) in times when I did an assistantship with Ludwig Binswanger.

Those Venetian days had been passed in the paths of spirituality by Franco Basaglia by reading his work with Scritti (1), especially the part named "Dalla Psichiatria Fenomenologica all'Esperienza di Gorizia".

I remembered that Franco Basaglia had affirmed in that unforgettable trip that the Daseinsanalyse, in which he attempted to interpret the incomprehensible world of the schizophrenic, had given end to the psychiatric nosology.

Ludwig Binswanger to create that interpretive system, had broken the "Vest of Formal Force" of the Classifying nomination in psychiatry releasing madness as a resource of infinite creativity: he discovered, for instance, in a catatonic schizophrenic the ετ δσζ husserlian of things that are terrifying; in a manic-depressive the Stimmung - the "humor" or "climate"-, of the celebration of death.

Infinite creativity: new categories of time and space, of the vigil and the dream, Olympic act of wounding of reality, discovery of disconcerting human dimensions: madness was an orphic fountain of knowledge.

The philosophical anthropology had taken the sickness of the Hippocratic signal of the extraordinary, of the accidental, to convert it in an ontologic category unnatural to man as transcendence and the word, with an arcane sense; destined to the deepest metaphysical meditation. Even more, the madness lost its horror and strangeness and transformed its adoration of philosophical knowledge.

Its hidden message and relevance was the creator of "dell'esperienza de Gorizia" in what Franco Basaglia assumed madness as priesthood and veneration of mystery.

Chased obsessively by a "maschera de la malattia" or the plague, I visited that afternoon in St. Michele in Isola, to meet an ancient Venetian ritual, Ezra Pound's tomb, "il miglior fabbro", the great maker of Thomas Stearns Eliot (2), who keeps silently the enigma of the Sibilia de Cumas:

> Once upon a time, I saw with my own eyes the Sibila de Cumas hung in a bubble. When the children asked her:Sibila: 'what do you want'? She answered them:'I want to die'
>
> This afternoon, I understood that only the madness damages the threshold of death...
>
> That is why for this return to metaphysics of madness is necessary to disregard its τ εκνε from the age of reason and asylums de Themis where. lives...

Without this introduction it would have been impossible to search out the baroque tragedy in times of the Inquisition in the Rio de la Plata Area, in which all personages are marked with an incomprehensible destiny, and where judges, tormentors and martyrs were trapped with the most incredible passion.

D. Emanvelle Tesavro (3) established in "Il Cannochiale Aristotelico O Sia Idea delle Argvtezze Heroiche", that this Argvtezza is a ... "trace of the Divine in the human soul".

He determined several forms of his "acuteness" in nature and man.

The human acuteness is proper to the "Ingegnosi", to the "furiosi" or violent and to the wisemen or "Esercitati".

In the furor is found significant alteration of the mind and, we find three entities: Passiono, Afflato and Pazzia.

This view of the acuteness where are met the passion, the divine enthusiasm of Orpheus, Hesiod, Homer... and madness brings the necessary categories to support our thesis, which has a reflection of the Latin American Coda in the revolution of 16th and 17th centuries in the west and should be introduced to the general dialectic of classicism and mannerism, explained by Ernst Robert Curtius (4) in which madness has a transcendental sense.

Ernst Curtius used the word mannerism to designate with a scientific term, all literary styles opposed to classic, so mannerism becomes a dialectic constant at all times.

We use the situation to point out madness as a figure of the gnomic forms of the creation process, without it, we would only have petrifaction and death.

In this dialectic movement through a negative process, we find non-classic variants with original structure.

The Latin American passion obtained dialectic forms in 16th and 17th centuries and faced the European mannerism in a transitional phase of new-classic post-renaissance and it is what we see in the circle of Inquisition of the River Plate Area. For instance, painful and changeable figures. A group of Cryptojewish messiahs, bizarre saints, heretic monks, Negro rebels, death's readers, aboriginal roots', Africans, Semitics and Celts.

A baroque tragedy that invites us to a game of horror and sadness. A baroque structure is like a deformed pearl whose irregularity gives it an extraordinary color - a gem with stains and warts - a skilled lecture; Erasmo, the crocodile is not so, but a tree or a rock; useless silogisms - in celarent aut baroco -; pilgrim toughness strange and irregular; heroic dreadfulness but unnecessary; a representation of effects without causes, a subjective disorder... In general, a drama of passion with ontologic revelations...

What was in common among judges, heretics and tormentors? Perhaps, the necessity of belonging to a furious hounds' pack (5) with a present feeling of death.

The reading of this topic of the Inquisition does not seem to make any sense at all, unless we read "Inquisition and the Spanish" by Juan Antonio Llorente* (6) compared with the English version of 1823 which sharpens its edges and hyperbolizes its critical references.

The presence of General Inquisitors from Spain was constituted on February 11, 1482, with Friar Alfonso de Celerian appointed as General Inquisitor of Spain by Pope Sixtus VI. In 1483, Friar Alfonso was replaced by Friar Tomas de Torquemada, who created the Supreme Council of the Holy and General Inquisition to Rule our America. Felipe II formed the Tribunal of the Holy Office in America on January 25, 1569.

The Tribunal of the Holy Office in Peru was proclaimed on January 29, 1570, and finished its period on September 18, 1820.

Cap. Manuel Frias proposed the creation of the Tribunal of the Inquisition in Port of Buenos Aires, city of La Trinidad, Rio de la Plata and letters to the King from the Attorney of the Audience of the Plata in 1636. In spite of all this that Tribunal was not created, fortunately.

Subject to the proclamation on January 29, 1570, our Inquisition was managed through delegates, which made the work quite twisted. Processes, inquisitorial letters, memorandums, references, edicts, requirements, chronicles, commentaries as examples of the "Hub of Inquisition", in the

---

* Llorente, J.A. (1758-1823) - The Inquisition and the Spanish, prolog and notes by Valentina Fernandez Vargas, 2nd. Ed. Madrid, Editorial Ciencia Nueva, 1967.

Llorenta, J.A. A Critical History of the Inquisition in Spain, from period of its establishment y Ferdinand V to the reign of Ferdinand VII, composed from original documents of Archives of the Supreme Council of the Inquisition and from those of subordinate tribunals of the Holy Office.
With an introduction by Gabriel H. Lovett/English ed. 1823/Williamstown, Mass., J Lilburne, 1867.

castle of Simancas located in Spain. Here is where the General Archive of the kingdom was used. We have worked there and the historical archives of Lima and also in the Archbishopric's, in the Tecuman's, Santiago del Estero y corrientes, where we found three folios unknown to date in the Archives of the Archbishopric in the Archdiocese of Cordoba strange horror's book of the Latin Witchcraft, with the name of Offices of the Holy Inquisition. The inquisition of Rio de la Plata, flourished in the period determined by Luis Alberto Sanchez, an American baroque writer, 1580-1680, which fell in progressive decadence and the witchcraft was substituted by a formal madness, pointed out by writer Jose Toribio Medina.

The themes found in this cannot be ordered in classes, orders, families, genders or species because in them, men and inequities were mixed up in noisy tornadoes; for instance , we find the Inquisitorial Marshall in Cochabamba, don Martin del Barco Centenera, who is creator of the Epic Poem "La Argentina", which has 10,720 verses classified in royal octaves and were called "hornillos de tiromento" (blast-furnaces of shooting) by Mr. Juan Maria Gutierrez, who was processed by the Inquisition, where he had served for years, with fourteen charges; "he was an indecent person who used to get drunk in the public houses, embracing a leather-bottle of wine".

On the other hand, Mr. Rodriguez de Guerrero, Secretary of the Governor of Tucuman was also processed because at the back of the holy sacrament he stabbed the Christ; Mr. Matias Delgado Flores, an envoy who took a prisoner, was enchained because of his apocalyptic madness, he wanted "to destroy convents and sow salt on their ruins"; there are some honored bishops like Friar Melchor Maldonado from Tucuman who was sued before the Holy Office, the Jesuit Loped de Mendoza because one day he was found very late in bed "with a joss-stick and a bunch of flowers on the table and also a bowl made of china full of colored water he used to spray on his face"; the sculptor Manuel de Couto, author of a "Holy Christ of our Cathedral" who was accused of "sitting on a saint's belly" by a metis servant girl who was being flattered by a Negro who wanted to save her from the insane artist...

The Inquisition as a madness transcended boundaries of death: Francisco de Aguirre was jailed twice for being a "blasphemer and quack" he died from loneliness in plain misery. Two years later the Governor of Chile, Felipe II ordered that the priest Manuel Nunez Magro, whose body already was buried, was be given to the justice to be burned in the corridor where were also burned the eleven accused of "complicidad grande" (great complicity) a crypto-jewish movement that wanted to establish the Jerusalem celeste (Heavenly Jerusalem) in Peru. Other members of the group of eleven were: Antonio de Espinosa the "great captain", Manuel Bautista Perez - the instructor of that beautiful dream -; the crazy Juan Rodriguez de Silva, affected from that sickness in prisons that was described in the modern times by S. Ganser; Tome Cuaresma, who asked for mercy, and the other condemned person: Diego Maldonado de Silva, the "statue of an extravagant", already dead, who was burned with the other martyrs in the Auto de Fe in 1639.

In accordance with the style of centuries, not only the readers of this procession, but also those who listened to its reading, who lived in times of Inquisition in Rio de la Plata, would have used St. Benedict's scapulary, which was made of coarse woolen fabric stained with yellow covering the whole body and knees, also stained with red crosses, bust in flames and vertical fires.

On their heads would be placed conic hats made of pasted paper, 836 mm high, with snakes and frogs painted and a very long tail, to mean the tortuous sophistication of our doctrines.

Many would have the witch's rope around their neck.

I. So, let us light first, the green candle of illuminations to treat the cryptojewish mechanisms: the bizarre sanctity; and the heresy of monks in XVI, XVII and XVIII centuries, chapter in our land of revolutions of the δαιμσεζ (demons) that we have mentioned and that appear in the European Renaissance as a presence of ancient gods who were exiled from a hidden and millennial tradition.

It would be necessary for many writers to be able to treat these themes in an exact way, but using the methods of ideographic models we will symbolize each type through examples in the particular which give us the contents of the general.

The history writer Toribio Medina (7,8,9) treated the passion of bachelor Francisco Maldonado de Silva, native of San Miguel city, Province of Tucuman "destos reinos del Piru", resident of City of Conception, kingdom of Chile, surgeon, son of the lawyer Diego Nunez de Silva, Portuguese doctor, brother of Diego de Silva reconciled for the Holy Office as "Heli Nazareo indigno del Dios de Israel"... He wondered if he were crazy or a martyr.

The answer is very simple: he was wonderfully crazy and a martyr as well.

Heli Nazareo substituted an orthodox fierce Catholicism for a holy messianic delirium in which he considered himself as one of the chosen "Two tribes of Israel were kept in paradise, expecting the world ending in which god joined them together and also multiplied".

He attempted to convert and save his sisters, but Felipa and Isabel Maldonado de Silva accused him before the Marshall of the Holy Office in Santiago taking him as a prisoner to City of Conception in Chile on "April 29, 1627 and jailed in the convent of Santo Domingo".

For action on October 12, 1627, came to the Holy Office: Father Jesuit Andres Hernandez rector of the college of his order Guamanga, and of the Major of St. Paul in Lima; Monk Luis de Bilbao, Doctor Pedro de Ortega, author of the Dictionary Historic-Bibliographic of Peru; Monk Alonso Briseno, an investigator from Ionnanis Scoti Doctoris Subtilis... with them he kept theological polemics, supported on the "illuminating power of its delirium" without any rectification of properties.

Bachelor Francisco Maldonado de Silva fasted for eighty days... "he got so weak that he could not even turn around in bed and only showing skin and bones and that very ulcerated, he asked for new advocates without any good result".

The prisoner collected corn cob's leaves and made a rope, "then he used it to escape through the window and went to other prisons nearby and persuaded the prisoners to follow his law... and he gave them letters to be delivered to Rome's synagogue when released from Inquisition".

He fasted so much that he got deaf, in his condition was celebrated the Auto de Fe on January 23, 1639, in Lima.

He was in jail for twelve years, that was not long enough to break the illuminations of his delirium... the tortures he suffered twisted his body and changed him to a bunch of "bones covered by skin, but his conviction remained the same".

The Jewish Boleslao Lewin (10) advises to read the books of the Lawyer Fernando de Montesinos about the "Auto de Fe celebrated in Lima on January 23, 1639; Tribunal of the Holy Office of Inquisition, the kingdoms of Peru, Chile, Paraguay and Tucuman" edited in Madrid by Imprenta del Reyno, 1640, to understand the sinister baroquism of our Inquisition.

From the text Tribunal of the Holy Office of Inquisition, I have rescued two paragraphs:

> Two Autos de Fe, the major have been celebrated in America. The one was made God the first Inquisitor, a) opposing to the Apostasy of Adam and Eve, the Theater of Paradise (Probably the opinion that brought him to Earth). b) On Sunday three days after the man was created. c) other V.S. on January 23d, 103 years after was found Peru. In the first God punished two heads, that infected the human race. In the Second V.S. relaxed two rabbis that taught the Apostasy and dead Law to many. That motivated from an apple, this from another one, with the difference that there the apple caused the loss of Adam's faith. d) And here he got to purify himself and twisting himself. The sad accent of Adam's apple in happiness..."
> Proverb of the Apple of Peru...

Curiously, the doctrine of Paradise in America, was defended by the Crypto-jewish Mr. Antonio de Leon Pinelo (11) who did not bite "the black apple of Peru".

He walked many times on the road to Lima de la Plaza de Armas, where there took place the Auto de Fe on January 23, 1639. From the street by the place and the bridge across the Rimac River to the church of the helpless and from the St. Lazarus street to the Pedregal where bachelor Francisco Maldonado de Silva was burned. In this pilgrimage, I have seen the sad figure of the martyr with his eyes twisted, deaf to everything but his delirium with his beard falling to his waist, erect and cadaverous with the amazing rightness of his infinite scriptures hanging from his neck converted in to a torch of marvelous madness.

That day at 3:00 PM, in the Auto de Fe when Diego Maldonado de Silva was condemned and released from secular justice to be condemned to be burned together with the Eleven cryptojewish of the "Complicidad grande". He provoked a strong wind to the curtain in the stage, so "God of Israel could see him face to face from heaven".

Moses once incinerated 23,000 heretics who adored the Golden Calf; Jose Maria Ramos Mejia (12) recalls in La Locura en la historia (Madness in the History) that in LX of Leviticus it is determined that "Man or woman possessed by Phiton or by the spirit of Divinity, shall be condemned to death.." The history of intolerance murder is immense and seems to be natural to man, but the baroquism in our Inquisition is hardly comparable.

That style accentuates the "coincidentia oppositorum" of his martyrdom, with the imposition condemning the excessive and bizarre religion of Cordoba de Tucumán, of the "holy order of the glorious patriarch San Augustin, the name of Anjela Carranza who for reasons of veneration was called mother Anjela who vainly named herself Anjela of God"

In 1665 she used to frequent temples and Holy Sacrament in Lima, with frenzy...

> She was in the tricked perception of mortals, the saint of this century, the wonder of this world, the mistress of the mystics, the lawyer of the people; miracles, ecstasies, rapes, intelligences and revelations, heaven was abridged in that woman. Courier of glory and for a new gender of sacred post office, took and brought from heaven answers and divine couriers...
>
> In fifteen years she wrote fifteen books of 54 notebooks, with more than 7500 pages Mistress and doctor of doctors. Among the revelations Sister Anjela had had, was one the Indian Nicolas de Aillon, or Nicolas of God, He had risen to heaven just after his death, accompanied by Jesus Christ and many spirits that had been released from purgatory, and they enjoyed the same glory as King David. Aillon was a tailor from Chiclaup, who had died in Lima with a reputation as a lamb of god in November 7, 1677. His woman Maria Jacinta de la Santisima Trinidad, negotiated before the Archbishop the sanctity of her husband, and she offered as a testimony her uncorrupted body.

When the Inquisition condemned Anjela Carranza to forswear of improper gaity and 5 years of severe retreat for a "prodigy of lies, fictions and ridiculous vanities seismic propositions, relaxive customs (11) and all type of insults", printed edicts were arranged to be given to the tribunal nine days after publication, "bills, rosaries, medals, bells, cowbells, swords, handkerchiefs, bandages with her blood, pieces of her skirt, nails, hair, scripts..." So many objects were collected that a complete room was full of them.

I am sure that it won't be boring the eternity of King David with a selection of mannerists like Nicolas de Dios y Anjela Carranza with whom we open the black door of the Apostasy.

We find the Dionisiac epidemic of the "solicitor" monks of St. Michael of Tucuman who between 16th to 17th centuries, preached in their confessional box the heresy of the illuminated, by which the act of love with them not only did not condemn but was a road of salvation.

There was also a multitude of "tormentors of Christ" not only of Portuguese gathered in Tucuman, but also including among them: Monk Diego de Lisboa as a suspect, Fernando Arias Ugarte a majordomo and confessor of the Archbishop of Lima and father of the talented writer Diego de Le—n Pinelo.

The funny Burguillos, famous in the chronicles of Lima, saw him entering the cathedral, taking with him a skirt to the Archbishop saying: "even if you get stuck to your tail, the Inquisition will take it out".

The heretical corruption of the sermons was almost worth the condemnation of the demented Franciscan, Monk Juan de Arregui, who in a homily of the Octave of the Virgin affirmed that "Maria was the white mare of Rua in which walked the holy sacrament" adding that "the gospels were roped horses".

The sermons of father Arregui were so picturesque that they attracted a crowd "obscene and vociferous" who listened to them in the church of the Convent of the Franciscan in Buenos Aires, which was considered scandalous by the Marshall Inquisitor Jorge Antonio Melendez de Figueroa, who could not light the fireplace because of the discourse considered a false rhetoric of innocent demented metaphors.

The 17th century marked the progressive end of the Inquisition with the birth of the new classicism and the enlightenment, it was abolished by the courts of Fernando VII. It disappeared completely on September 18, 1820.

Before it had requisitioned the library of Bishop Azamor that profiled the lectures of those of his class: French edition of the Paradise Lost of Milton; the letter of Jewish to Voltaire; the Social Contract of Rousseau; the Dictionary of Bayle... Francomasonry had entered into Rio de la Plata and excited the passion of militaries and intellectuals.

In the 19th century the heretic rebellion of the Bishop of Currents don Benito de la Lue y Riega took place, against the inquisitor don Juan Jose de Arce, blocking the reading of the edicts of faith and anathema.

I have walked through the memories of the bishop, "like the most imprudent madman we have got from the other side of the ocean" that slept under the bed so as not to be hurt by moon's rays and put his head in tubs of cold water until up ached, to defeat his heretical ideas, and committed the most unimaginable irreverences, boasting of an extreme reculturisation which characterized our Inquisition.

II. Let us put out the green candle of iniquity to deal with necromants who read the death of tradition of Celts, Semitics, blacks and aboriginals.

In the ruins of ancient Santa Fe (13), exists the most firm testimonies regarding Mediterranean witchcraft in our America, kept in a Crypt, we find: La higa (Scorn), the twitching hand, which means the Jewish word of three letters that exorcises the eye illness. Treated by St. Tomas de Aquino and the Marques Enrique Villena and caused, according to the Talmud, ninety nine out of one hundred deaths; the Bezoar Stone which was taken from America to the Monastery of San Jeronimo de Yuste to cure the melancholy of Carlos V; pellets made of colored glass and mica leaves; handbells against lighting, perforated coins and talismans; clover with four leaves; amulets from animals; representations of snakes; marine shells and many other mixed symbols of exorcism, proper to black and aboriginal people.

The great models of witchcraft from Lima: Ana Maria de Contreras, a mulatto slave killed by lighting and she became clairvoyant; Ana de Campos, metis from Guamanga, neighbour of Cuzco to whom the evil one visited wearing a grey calf's dress; Mrs. Beatriz Vandera, to whom appeared a monkey with a long tail; and Mrs. Estefania Ramirez de Meneses, who appeared in the Autos with a green candle in her hand, a rope around her neck and was condemned to be whipped and exiled: it was subject to a search in our country and excited to passion of psychiatrists in the beginning of century.

Jose Ingenieros wrote an essay in the Medical Week of February 12, 1920 (14); the texts of the History writer from Tucuman José López Manián (15,16) about the witch Luisa Gonzalez India and Pascula India. Andres Figueroa wrote about Lucrecia India; Anibal Ponce (17) treated the "psychopathology of Retreat" using as a reference the manuscripts of Swiss Cecilia Ve, studied by Flournoy and judged as a mere verbalism, the interpretation of Sigmund Freud (18) made about totem and taboo in the French translation of Jankélévitch.

The Tecuman doctor Emilio Catalán (19,20) whose thesis about Systematized Madness (5), in 1914 gives us a reflective knowledge about the classification of delirium and reminds us that the worse tormentor of witchcraft in Rio de la Plata was the governor of Tucuman, Juan Ramirez de Velazco, who lit in the 16th century more bonfires than absolutions, than the Inquisition did in all American history. He judged India Ana, Magdalena India, Lucrecia India and especially Ynes Negra "who put wind in the head" of wife of Cap. Francisco de Luna and Cardenas.

We have added to this collection the lecture in three folios of the Holy Office of Inquisition from the Archives of the Archdiocese of Cordoba.

The witches of MacBeth, the abominable furies of the Caprices of Goya, the Montiela de Miguel de Cervantes (21), who died because Camacha transformed her children into dogs, find their parallels in the magical Argentinean baroque.

From these books of great value for the histography of the Inquisition, I have only picked some anecdotes to be used as models of ethnic witchcraft of Rio de la Plata whose tradition is Mediterranean, Celtic, African and Aboriginal.

Among them, the one from a confessional box of a women: Juan Pablo Villalba is accused by his wife Mrs. Maria de Hara and his sister Isabel, of blasphemy because he damned God, his soul, birthday, holy sacraments, the whole creation and he practiced witchcraft on tombs.

Holding a coral in his left hand, he produced the medusian death, but with his right hand he resuscitated the dead.

The hand of the courtly representative of "Arte Cisoria" (22,23) held a venemous coral serpent. The coral is a water tree, a species of axis mundi, an element of the Neptunian Cosmogonies, of Medusa's blood: animal, vegetable and mineral.

The African witchcraft, swords and worms, terrified and parasitical earth, dark and underground symbol of rottenness, monsters: Captain Negro "the worst witch of the world" and

Jose Angola de Nacion, a cook of the Fathers of the Company of Jesus in Cordóba del Tucuman.

The other witchcrafts... the chicken wool's to filter damage... the Petronela de los Molena's with a partridge on the chest until the bird died to incarnate evil... the black musician's with the evil music... All of them inspired in the fear of Cordoba del Tucuman.

Madness goes beyond manneristic (24, 25 ,26, 27) creativity and forms structures which are frozen within a living myth.

We have put our tribute shield of the Inquisition - a green cross on a black field, and olives branch at the right and a sword at the left - underneath the Moses burning bush and on the back the cross of Santo Domingo as being from Rio de la Plata, the expression of the cruel baroque. The European Mannerism of the counterreformation reached the American dimensions with a dialectic spiral of classicism - mannerism to address total madness.

We have developed briefly a fantastic design of the Rio de Plata's "delegation".

Expressive violences and desperate fights to trap world's secrets, through a pathetic labyrinth of God, where only the fright is beautiful and atrocious.

The Saturnian melancholy interrupts the old pages of the chronicles to testify about the convulsive beauty, amazing pulvarization of the damned, a paranoiac, serpentinean and torturous superdimensional.

It is intrinsic to the baroque that certain classicism is erected with the dialectic antimony of design. The baroque reaches its terrifying essence with the negation of the negation, confusion and extravaganza, violation of rules and caprices in spite of the arificial structure of cardboard walls, of shattered grapevines and the sight of God's image in our martyrs and a sketch of the area surrounding the notion of the unlimited and infinite.

A tragedy of fury, Latin term of the sacred mania of Greeks, that awakened the ages.

References

1. Basaglia, F.; Scritti, I. - 1953-1968, Della psichiatria fenomenologica all'esperienza di Gorizia, A cura di Franca Ongaro Basaglia. Torino, Giulio Inaudi, 1981.

2. Eliot, T.S. - The Waste Land (1922) En: T. S. Eliot, The Complete Poems and Plays of. London, Faber and Faber, 1960.

3. Tesuaro, E. - II Cannochiala Aristotelico... dal Conte D. Emanvuele Tesavro. In Veneti Presso Paolo Baglioni, M. D.C. LXXIV.

4. Curtius, E. R. - Europäische Literatur und lateinische Mittelalter. Bern. A. Francke AG Verlag, 1948.

5. Canetti, E. - Masse und Macht. Hamburg, Classen Verlag, 1960.

6. Llorente, J. A. - Histoire critique de l'Inquisition d'Espagne. (Trad. Alexis Pellier). Paris, Treuttel et Wurtz, 1817-1818.

7. Medina, J. T. - Historia del Tribuna de la Inquisici—n de Lima (1569-1820). Pr—logo de Marcel Bataillon. Santiago de Chile, Fondo Hist—rico y Bibliográfico J. Medina, 1956.

8. Medina, J. T. - Historia del Tribunal del Santo Oficio de la Inquisici—n en Chile. Pr—logo de Aniceto Almeyda. Santiago de Chile, Fondo Hist—rico y Geográfico J. T. Medina 1952.

9. Medina, J. T. - El Tribunal del Santo Oficio de la Inquisici—n en las Provincias del Plata. Santiago de Chile, Imprenta Elzeviriana, 1899.

10. Leon, B. - El Santo Oficio en América. Buenos Aires, Sociedad Hebraica Argentina, 1950.

11. Leon Pinelo, A. de - El Paraiso en el Nuevo Mundo, Comentario Apologético, Historia Natural y Peregrina de las Islas Occidentales, Yslas y Tierra Firme del Mar Océano. Por el licenciado D. Antonio de León Pinelo, Del Consejo de S. M. y su oydor en la Casa de Contratación a las Yndias que reside en las Ciudad de Sevilla. Ano de MDCLVI Copiado por Dn. Josef Sobrino y Manxon, Oficial de la Contratacion a Yndias en Cádiz. Ano de 1779.

12. Ramos Mejia, J. M. - La Locura en la Historia. Con una introducción de Paul Groussac, Buenos Aires, Talleres Gráficos Argentinos, L. J. Rosso, 1933.

13. Zapata Gollan, A. - Supersticiones y amuletos. Santa Fe, Ministerio de Educación y Cultura. Deparamento de Estudios Coloniales, Segunda Epoca Nro. 1, 1960.

14. Ingenieros, J. - Locura y brujería en la sociedad colonial. En: La Semana Médica. Buenos Aires, febrero 12 de 1920, págs. 220-233.

15. Lopez Manan, J. - La prueba testimonial en la supercheria, justicia criminal tucumana en el siglo XVIII. En: J. López Manán, Tucumán Antiguo. Buenos Aires, Colección del Sesquicentenario de la Independencia Argentina. Universidad Nacional de Tucumán, 1916.

16. Lopez Manan, J. - Justicia criminal tucumana en el siglo XVIII. Suplicio de una bruja. En: Archivos de Psiquiatria y Criminologia aplicadas a las Ciencias Afines. Ano III, enero-febrero 1904, págs. 602-614.

17. Ponce, A. - Psicopatología del Conjuro. Revista de Filosofia, Ano XI, Nro. 4, julio de 1925, págs. 275-289.

18. Freud, S. - Totem et Tabou. Traduction S. Jankélévitch. Paris, Bibliothèque Scientifique, 1923.

19. Catalan, E. - Estudio clinico sobre las locuras sistematizadas, persecutorias, misticas, eróticas. (Tesis), Buenos Aires, Libreria "Las Ciencias", 1914.

20. Catalan, E. - La brujeria penada con la hoguera en el Tucumán Colonial. Revista de Filosof'a. Ano XII, Nro. 3, 1926, págs. 461-469.

21. Lanuza, J. L. - Las Brujas de Cervantes. Buenos Aires, Academia Argentina de Letras, 1973.

22. Villena E. de Aragon, Marques de, - Arte Cisoria. Prepar— el texto Federico Carlos Sainz de Robles. Madrid, Espasa-Calpe, 1967.

23. Villena, E. de Aragon, Marques de, - "Tres tratados: II. Tratado de Alojamiento". Revue Hispanique, T. XLI, 1917, págs. 182-197.

24. Hocke, G. R. - Die Welt als Labyrinth Manier und Manie in der europáischen Kunst. Hanburg, Rowohlt Taschenbuch Verlag GmbH, 1957.

25. Hocke, G. R. - Manierismus in der Literatur Sprach-Alchimie und esoterische Kombinationskunst. Hamburg, Rowohlt Taschenbuch Verlag GmbH, 1957.

26. Sypher, W. - Four States of Renaissance Style; Transformation in Art and Literature, 1400-1700, Garden City, N.J. Doubleday, 1955.

27. Wolfflin, H. - Renaissance and Baroque. Translated by Kathrin, with an Introduction by Peter Murray. Ithaca, N. Y. Cornell University Press, 1966.

Frenzies of Possession by the Fox of Japan (or Frenzy by Kitsune-Tsuki)

F. Furukawa and M. Bourgeois

Summary: The frenzies of possession by the 'fox' (Kitsune-Tsuki) - when examined are actually in the animist context of Shintoism - either the frenzies of sorcery by tormenting malevolence descendent from the ancient healers of the 'fox' (Mochi-Suji), or the frenzies of simple possession. This alopecanthropy appears to differ from the cases of European zoanthropy (example: lycanthropy) by the absence of bodily transformation. It brings together the demonopathic and relieves varied psychopathological states.

Proposed is a review of literature and six observations - of this original syndrome narrowly linked to Japanese culture and its traditional beliefs.

THE FRENZY OF POSSESSION BY THE 'FOX' or the frenzy of Kitsune-Tsuki represents an original psychiatric syndrome, proper to Japan where its the best known of frenzies of animal possession. It differs from the cases of European zoanthropy in that, in the specific case of the animal possessor (the fox), is a demon in the ancient sense of genius or divinity. (In the following of this account when we speak of the fox we must understand we mean the soul or the spirit of the fox).

The importance of the fox in Japanese mentality comes from its association with the Shintoist god of prosperity: Inari. Two different psychiatric states are described under the term frenzy by Kitsune-Tsuki:

1.- The possession by the fox which is a frenzy of sorcery

2.- The frenzy of simple possession by the fox

These frenzies of animal possession have been considered for a long time as anachronic. The first type - enchantment by the fox - has already disappeared. The frenzy of simple possession can already be observed in a sporadic manner but is already in the course of disappearing. We will present these different pictures with some observations, in stressing the differences with the cases of European zoanthropy. First we make a brief cultural and religious reminder to place Shintoism and above all the fox, his cult and his superstition in traditional Japanese mentality, according to the Ishizuka (1959) and Kondo (1978) ethnologies.

The Superstition of the Fox and Shintoism

Shinto (literally the Road or Teaching of the gods) or Shintoism, was the national religion of Japan, prior to the introduction of Buddhism (6th century). The ancient Shinto consisted of a group of beliefs and animistic rites without dogma, without sacred writings, without a known founder. This polytheist religion has a considerable number of divinities (Kami). Since the 14th century Shinto, which views the emperor as a representative of the gods, was transformed into a national religion. It was officially separated from the state in 1946, although Shinto remains influential.

In this traditional animist religion, ill will can render the souls of the living and the dead malignant (Akuryo or Mono-Noke) and makes them play a demonic role. But Shintoism is not black and white. The gods can either be evil or favourable. When they are revered by offerings, they bestow and bless the faithful. If we neglect them they get revenge and make havoc: accidents, poverty, illnesses, and calamities strike the unfaithful. They must then multiply their prayers and offerings. We can thus maintain the benevolent character of the divinity or even reconcile with the malevolent demonic divinities.

The fox (Kitsune) is an intelligent animal, sly and prudent. For the Japanese, this is not only an animal creature, a zoological existence, its also a spiritual being, a force, a genius. The ancient Japanese dreaded it as a worried creature, malevolent, frightening, like a diabolic monster. Always honored by prayers and offerings, we can placate its beneficent part and make it an amicable divinity. Frequently observed near rice fields, the fox being celebrated and considered as a heralding god and god of cereals: Inari (literally: he who brings rice). Thus the vassal of Inari, is often represented with seven tails, symbolizing the magical force. Really the spirit of the fox does not necessarily take the form of a fox (thus a weasel that runs around the house could be considered as being the fox, the same goes for objects, for men, etc...)

Under the influence of Buddhism, particularly in the sect of sorcery (Mikkyo), introduced to Japan in the 8th century, Inari changed in function. He became the god of prosperity. The Mikkyo sect had among its magical proceedings the method of invocation of Dakini (god of Indian origin) to ask for prosperity. Dakini is also accompanied by the fox and Inari is identified with Dakini. The fox is thus respected as he who brings happiness. By the temples of Inari the healers belong to the influence of the fox; they practiced divination, invocation and exorcisms with the mediation of the fox. The objects of this practice are, for example bamboo, or any object where the spirit of the fox could lodge.

Beginning in the 18th century the cultural level of the people was high enough so that it's life did not depend on the magical force of the fox. There was a recoil from animism. One problem persisted however: the foxes inherited by the descendants of healers remained without use, in half-pay of some sort. The immaterial beings (that can lodge anywhere) are aroused and become frightening forces. Abandoned without prayers or offerings they become demonic and malfeasant. Up until 1950 some families continued to practice the cult of the fox in their homes. The healers continued to borrow their power from the fox.

The expression Kitsune-Tsuki (possessed by the fox) is frequently used since this era. It does not necessarily signify the classic picture of possession. It can designate a simple confused state. It became also a sort of metaphor to designate and explain, within the limits of humour, a failure or a disagreement, but with the persistence of a deep superstitious belief. A certain worry always remains present.

The small gods sometimes escape to the domination of their patron and play bad tricks. It is the same for the fox and the healers. People fear that they may escape and become malfeasant. The descendants of the healers are called Mochi-Suji or Kitsune-Mochi. Mochi-Suji designates a family who, from generation to generation, tames the fox and uses his spiritual force. We believe that this family can avenge whoever wrongs them in possessing them with the fox. This superstition give rise to the frenzy of possession by the fox, who is in the frenzy form of sorcery. This type of frenzy is localized and epidemic.

Intrigues were brought by the ethnologist, Ishizuka (1959) from 1948 to 1955 when permitted to geographically locate the Mochi-Suji superstition in Honshu, the principal island in the Japanese archipelago. Honshu was divided into 4 zones, each zone corresponding with one of the 4 phases of development of the Mochi-Suji superstition. This division was historically linked to the territorial extension of the ancient empire by the Yamato clan held by Shintoism in the third century. In the ancient frontier zone the belief in the fox stayed primitive. We can observe the belief in the fox in a part of the Kyu-Shu and Shi-Koku, the two other large islands in the south-west of Honshu, but we have less documents for these regions.

1- The region north-east of Honshu: the fox was revered. We put confidence in the healers who used the fox. Possession by the fox was not strongly dreaded for it could be controlled and used to divine ends, obtaining an oracle and even healing.

2- The region center - east of Honshu: the fox is almost abandoned. Sorcery by the fox is rare. The healers often earn their living in other professions. Rarely, when there were clients, did they practice sorcery. They were called, as were their descendants, Mochi-Suji, but were not necessarily dreaded or detested. According to the documents invoked by Ishizuka we can guess the sporadic apparitions of frenzy of possession by the fox as a form of frenzy of sorcery.

3- The region west of Honshu: There the fox is punished, mostly in the north half. We believe that the fox only protected the Mochi-Suji families. These Mochi-Suji families were aloof. The matrimonial union was honored with them, because they also became Mochi-Suji and that was a curse. They dreaded the resentment of the Mochi-Suji and their revenge by the fox. The healers practiced exorcisms against the fox. They did not belong to Mochi-Suji families. It is in this region that the frenzies of sorcery-possession by the fox are frequent. All the healers do not interpret sorcery by the fox. They do not practice all their exorcisms by the fox. In the south half of the west region there were certain frenzies of possession by the divine dog.

4- The region center - west of Honshu: They did not know troubles. In the temples of Inari, the fox always remained calm.

The Frenzy of Sorcery - Possession by the Fox in San-in Region

Literature reveals that the frenzies of possession by the fox were often evoked for 200 years (Shinfuku 1959, Ishizuka 1959, Miyamoto 1979, Oda 1981). But the frenzy of possession that the manifestation of sorcery was relatively localized to the region west of Honshu and more particularly in the north half of San-In. Shinfuku (1959), pupil of Morita, did the clinical study of this type of frenzy. He considers it as a reactional psychosis and distinguishes it from another frenzy of Kitsune-Tsuki: The phenomenon of possession by the fox can be seen in the diverse endogenous or exogenous psychoses, but the true frenzy of possession by the fox is a linked psychosis: be it the superstitious belief or the suggestion that Mochi-Suji can provoke the possession of someone by the fox, or the exorcism to chase the fox who possesses a subject (exorcism practiced by a healer). He divides these cases into 3 subtypes:

1) Original subtype

He remembers the primitive reactions such as Arctic hysteria. Two observations illustrate this type:

Observation no. 1 (Shinfuku, 1959)

Woman of 33 years. One day cut down a tree to make logs. Learns afterwards that this tree was property of a Mochi-Suji family. As soon as she realizes this her hands start to tremble. She becomes dizzy and something ridiculous begins running in her stomach. She becomes a gossip and sings songs. Finally she enters a state of possession.

Observation no.2 (Shinfuku, 1959)

Woman of 20 years. Succeeds at getting a job. Her unhappy competitor for this job is of the Mochi-Suji family. As soon as she finds this out, her arms and legs become paralyzed. During the night she sees and hears the fox. She repeats that her four limbs cannot move because she is possessed by the fox. During the exorcism, the change in personality is evident; she speaks like the fox.

In this sub-type, the fear of the Mochi-Suji provokes the possession by the fox arising in certain circumstances, to the occasion of everyday events like for example summoning one of the members of the Mochi-Suji to pay his debts, meeting him when we are (too?) well dressed, not inviting him for a meal, or having more money than usual. The majority of the victims were women, usually uncultivated. This subtype of frenzy has a greater tendency than others to repeat itself. It is more specific in this region but psychiatrists saw little of it because these were healers who habitually took care of them. The accounts of Shinfuku are thus based on the accounts of healers. While subtype 1 belongs to reactions of fright, the subtypes 2 and 3 appear after a period of latency, with ruminations of the patient concerning a personal illness, or that of one close, financial worries, child delinquency, etc., to the occasion of an emotional decompensation the subject falls into a frenzy of sorcery-possession by the fox. In subtype 2 it is the healer consulted that suggests to the sick person that he is a victim of sorcery-possession of the fox. In subtype 3, the sick person discovers himself the explanation coming from the fear of the Mochi-Suji.

2) Subtypes 2 & 3

They were not analyzed separately. We come from seeing that it is the mechanism of appearance that distinguishes them (suggestion by a third or auto-suggestion) and not the clinic. Shinfuku insisted on the fact that we could not clearly distinguish the clinical pictures one from the other. He always states that in 24 cases cured in the neuro-psychiatric service at the University of Tottori (San-In region) in 7 years (1951-1957), 16 were type 2, and 8 were type 3. Here are two observations:

Observation No. 3 (Shinfuku, 1959)

Woman of 43 years. For a year has been frequenting the temple of Inari and makes invocations to cure her neuralgia. She finishes by saying: amid my cousins there is one possessed by the fox. She made me possessed by the fox because I show her no friendship. The fox is lodged in my body, and orders me to do various things. She tears up vegetables and throws them in a repetitive fashion saying that its the orders of the fox. In the same way she never goes to bed.

Observation no.4 (Shinfuku, 1959)

Woman of 36 years, of the timid and fearing type. Has had economic difficulties for several years. Suddenly one night she cries the fox has possessed her, and the Buddha has possessed her. Sometimes she cries, sometimes she laughs. Then she does violence to her family; she raises and lowers her arms in a repetitive fashion, eats her meals like a four legged animal, and says it's against her will that she acts like this.

For types 2 and 3 we see the same female prevalence (22 women out of 24 people or 92%) and a mediocre level of education. As for the level of religiousness, 4 subjects were believers, and 16 (of type 3) had become religious just before the appearance of symptoms. The age ranges from 16 to 67 years, most are middle age- 30-35 years - (17 out of 24, or 71%). The pre-morbid character is described as hysteric for 9 ill people, epileptic for 5, timid and fearing (oversensitive?) for 4, and schizoid for 3 subjects. The principal symptom was a personality change (Jinkaku-Henka) in 5 cases, the idea of possession in 21 cases, the idea of persecution for 6 cases, of influence in 5 cases, and finally 1 case of depersonalization. Ten of the ill suffered from hallucinations: somatic hallucinations (8 cases), verbal auditives (6 cases), visual (6 cases), psychic (1 case). One sick person was disoriented and 8 were agitated. The duration of the period of the state was not provided. The prognosis was favorable. Shinfuku states that among 16 ill people (3 after relapse) complete healing was reached. But 6 among them kept the belief that their illness was caused by the fox.

Among the possessed described by Shinfuku there is a clear distinction between the instigator of the possession (Mochi-Suji), the agent of the possession (the fox) and the victim of the possession (the ill person). We find the habitual component of the frenzy of sorcery is the accusation of a third person, who is responsible for the sorcery and persecution (Bourgeois, 1971). Very particular here is the intervention of the third element or person, the fox, as the carrier of witchery. We momentarily propose to designate this type of frenzy = possession by the fox as a frenzy of sorcery, or more simply = frenzy of sorcery possession by the fox.

The Frenzy of Simple Possession of the Fox

The other form of possession by the fox does not need the intervention of a third party. We can designate it as a simple frenzy of possession or a frenzy of simple possession by the fox. It's the fox himself in his original demonic dimension, not yet purified by the prayers that is responsible for the witchery. We already find descriptions of this type of frenzy in texts of the 9th century. For example a confused subject presents during an exorcism with personality changes and declares: " I am the fox: because I was killed by this man, I will possess him and kill him". The exorcism cannot prevent the fox from killing the possessed person (cited by Oda, 1981).

Actually, cases of this type of frenzy are described within the framework of a syndrome of possession by Yap (1960). For example, 5 out of 26 cases of possessed people described by Rhee (1961) were possessed by the fox or other animals. Out of 15 cases of Kuba (1973), one was possessed by the fox. Sato and colleagues. (1975) encountered 2 cases of possession by the fox in 2 years (1973-74). Seven out of 19 cases of Nishimura (1976) were possessed by the fox.

Here is an observation by Nishimura (1978):

Observation no. 5 (Nishimura, 1978)

Man of 47 years, married, municipal official. Born in a village in the north-east region of Honshu. No psychiatric antecedent in his family. Since the end of his primary studies he has been an official in his home town. He was married at 29 years and has two sons. When he was 42 there was a conflict between two unions of officials from his office. Almost all the members of his department belong to the opposite union as he did. He has a feeling of isolation. It results in a psychotic state with auditory and verbal hallucinations and frenzy of persecution whose essential theme is that his colleagues and his superior want to chase him out of office. Then his frenzy of persecution changes to a frenzy of jealousy: he believes his wife and one of his colleagues are in love and that his wife wants to replace him. At the end, he talks to his wife about his ideas and preoccupations. She is very surprised and thinks her husband is possessed by the fox. During these invocations and exorcisms, his symptoms momentarily disappear. One time with a very popular healer he finally shows the change in personality. During the exorcism he walks on all fours, cries out like an animal, jumps, falls. He momentarily loses consciousness. When he regains consciousness his symptoms have totally disappeared. But rapidly after going back to work he is again taken by the idea of possession. He suffers again from a feeling of isolation. He thinks "I am possessed by the fox. He torments my body. He makes me do diverse things. He makes me play. I see bizarre animals." His wife wants to bring him to the healer. But circumstances do not permit. The sick person is thus hospitalized where he receives the diagnosis of schizophrenia. A year and a half passes. He is transferred to a hospital near his home. There the doctors listen carefully to his complaints and his conviction of being possessed by the fox. Thanks to this he suddenly leaves his catatonic state and after six months of hospitalization shows a complete remission.

Finally, we present the case of a sick person who we knew and whose hospital records we obtained from 1982 to 1983. Schizophrenia was evolving for her since the age of 25, treated at Tokyo Women's Medical College. When her state got worse in August 1982, the service being complete, she was sent to Takao-Hoyo-In hospital.

Observation no. 6 (original, 1982-83)

Woman of 50 years, single. Born in a village in the center-west region of Honshu. Fourth in a sibline of six. Daughter of an employee. After leaving high school she continued to live with her parents with no fixed work (in Japan it is not rare that a woman remains without work in the family, up until marriage). Actually lived in Tokyo. No psychiatric antecedent in the family. Had schizophrenia since 1957 (25 years). She had already been hospitalized three times and appears to be in remission without chemotherapy when she had a relapse in August 1982. She became agitated, violent and aggressive towards her mother. She believes that the fox is transformed in her mother to torment her. She enters Takao-Hoyo-In hospital. She complains that six foxes have possessed her: "They talk to me in what seems to be human voices. They are lodged in my head, my shoulders and my stomach.". She often presents the attitude of trying to rid herself of snakes. These black snakes are under direction of the foxes. Under the orders of the foxes, the snakes penetrate her uterus. One night in an dreamlike state, she sees the snakes, is very scared and cannot enter her room. She says the foxes are about three cm. in size, in quasi-human form with pointed ears and short tails. She thinks they are of the male sex, because they asked her for her hand. Under neuroleptics the picture improves and she leaves the hospital in Sept. 1983.

In the 1970's, the frenzies of simple possession by the fox were frequent in the north-east region of Honshu (Sato 1975, Nishimura 1976). But this region has now reached phase 4 of Ishizuka. The healers who do not attribute the witchery to the fox have lost the confidence of the people (Nishimura 1978). But it did not have the Mochi-Suji family and the rapid elevation to the cultural level did not favor this notion of danger. The Japanese authors in general divided the clinical pictures of possession into three = reactionary picture, psychotic picture and dreamlike picture. Sometimes we employ the notions of Oesterreich = "dual diachronic personality" (hysteria), "dual synchronic personality" (schizophrenic + hysteric dissociation) and we add the state of dreams. Amid the 12 cases the authors (two cases of Rhee 1961, one case of Kuba 1973, eight cases of Nishimura 1976 and 1978, one personal case). There are eight women and four men. Six women and two men presented the change of personality (reactionary picture or "dual diachronic personality"). Except for one 24 year old sick person, the age of these sick people is between 40 and 67 years. three women and one man had the experience of dual synchronic personality or psychotic picture. The ages at the beginning of the illness are: 22, 25, 51 and 63 years. The dreamlike states were observed with a sick person of 32 years and one of 39 years. The diagnoses of the basic mental illnesses are: keen neurotic reactions, atypical neuroses, psychoses, schizophrenia and psychosis of invocation of Morita (1915).

Psychosis of Invocation of Morita (1915)
(Invocation Psychosis)

This pathology occurs on the occasion of the invocation of divinities and prayers to get rid of misfortune. According to Morita:

> It is a particular psychosis caused by the invocation (the prayer) or similar circumstances in which we can observe the personality change, and the appearance of religious and/or possession ideas. The duration is from a few days to a few months. Women are stricken more than men. The sick people are ignorant... The superstitious subjects, believing in possession, in religious punishments or spiritualism suddenly fall into this psychosis, when they are confronted with frightening events or a bodily illness that they consider strange. This psychosis appears at the time of prayer or exorcism... the clinical picture is ordinarily keen, sometimes subacute. When there is a change in personality, the illness transforms itself into a dead parent or child, into Buddha, or into the fox, and causes involuntary behavior. During the change in personality the conscience of the sick person is, quite clearly, profoundly altered. But in general, the memory is well preserved. In addition, because of the influenced syndrome, the sick person is often afraid, anguished, emotionally confused, agitated... the change of personality is a passenger, from a few minutes to dozens of minutes. Sometimes it repeats itself several times a day... in the intervals, the sick person shows discreet symptoms such as irritability, anxiety, or incoherence. The temporo-spatial orientation is usually preserved... after the experience of the change of personality, the patient might get a religious idea or an idea of possession. Certain patients might induce the change of personality to their pleasure by auto-suggestion... there are no hallucinations, other than rare cases of pseudo-hallucination... a change in environment is the best treatment... the differential diagnosis with dementia praecox and degenerative psychosis (paranoia) is essential. Dementia Praecox can in fact begin with identical symptoms and circumstances. The change in personality is the best diagnostic guiding mark... in the psychosis of invocation, the change in personality is, even if it appears catatonic, is composed of involuntary acts after auto-hypnosis... during inter-critical periods the diagnosis is made according to the affective state = fear, anxiety or perplexity. But it is sometimes difficult when the sick person is distracted from the outside world by religious ideas of possession... we cannot put this psychosis in another traditional frame such as the second state, affective confusion, neurasthenia, keen paranoia and expected neurosis... among the psychoses of invocation, we can find three forms: confused, stuporous and change of personality... and I include in this psychosis, the local cases of the frenzy of possession by the divine dog by the fox and other animals.

In fact, the question as to whether this psychosis is an entity or not, still remains open. Sometimes schizophrenia arises from this religious experience. Often, the clinical picture alone is not sufficient for the diagnosis, and we must consider the premorbid character, the age at the beginning, the sex, the circumstance of the appearance, etc. (Miyamoto 1979). Murakami describes a degenerative psychosis (paranoia) with a great reaction tendency (1979, cited by Miyamoto 1979). Ogino considers Morita's description as purely phenomenal. Miyamoto (1979) indicates that Morita wanted to isolate the reactionary frenzies of possession. The notion of invocation psychosis had a great influence on the descriptions of the frenzy of possession in Japan.

Comments

We have distinguished two forms of frenzy of possession by the fox, one - the frenzy of sorcery/ possession - was a passenger (for about two centuries) and has now disappeared. It appeared in a period of socio-cultural change where sorcery by the fox became socially less necessary. The other frenzy of possession, that we simply qualified, is founded on the superstition of the demonic fox, his intervention in an evil third person. The term alopecanthropy is used in the medical-psychiatric Japanese vocabulary to translate the popular word for frenzy of Kitsune-Tsuki. It was criticized by Miyamoto (1979) because it brought back the notion of zoanthropy. Our alopecanthropes do not have the idea of a transformation or of a metamorphosis into an animal. On the other hand, one of the alopecanthropes cited by Calmeil (1845) said: "I am seen in the form of a wolf: I walk on all fours, my limbs are covered with long hair." The fox comes to lodge himself in the human body. But the frenzy of possession by the fox is not zoopathic either. The fox uses his influence on the human spirit. In zoopathic possession the animals do not exert bodily influence. In this sense our last case (no. 6) is interesting. She attributes zoopathy to snakes controlled by foxes. It appears that these foxes have not completely lost their divinity: the sick person hesitates to name their sex. This alopecanthropy thus resembles a European demonopathic (but it presents as schizophrenia). Seglas (1985) described it in three forms: external demonopathy, internal demonopathy and true demonic obsession. In Japan we observe similar cases to external demonopathy and also internal demonopathy. But the change in personality indicates the difference with true demonic obsession. For Seglas "to true demonic obsession is fastened zoanthropy, lycanthropy, that in fact are only modalities"... the individual is transformed into a demon: but the demon embodies itself in an animal, the sick person has himself become the diabolical animal. The logic of animism does not need a certain complex procedure. We can say "the individual lodges in the diabolical soul; this soul is that of the fox, thus the sick person himself has become this diabolical animal." The substitution of the soul or the spirit is sufficient to make our zoanthropy. This explains why according to Oesterreich (1904), in Japan there were lots of cases of possession by animals (cited by Daiguji and colleagues, 1975). We suggest that the fox is not a devil or a Christian demon. The possessed do not feel guilty, on the contrary the European sick people who like a sick person of J. Delay "accuse themselves of abominable crimes; he killed his father and wanted to strangle his mother, he could do nothing but think and do wrong." The ideas of damnation (Melancholic) are not rare. Japan is the instigator of witchcraft of which it is accused.

For the psychopathology of the frenzy of possession in general, Ogino (1974) adopted the notion of 'downfalls of psychological strain' of Janet. Ogino thus indicates that in the clinical pictures we can recognize two types: reactionary and schizophrenic. In the reactionary type, the personality separation of principal-personality/accessory is complete. The ill person has a dual personality. In the schizophrenic type, the accessory personality is immersed in the principal personality. The sick person experiences hallucinations and a syndrome of influence. At a profound level of the downfall of psychic strain, we can observe a second state or a diachronic dual-personality, dream state, and catatonic state. At a less profound level, we can observe a dual synchronic personality and a paraphrenic picture. Miyamoto (1979) proposed, to explain the idea of schizophrenia of possession the notion of the enlargement of Moi (Ego-Enviterung). This enlargement is a process of the inclusion of others in the Moi and the identification to these other. The syndrome of possession is a means of evasion. The people who mistrust modern scientific culture ask for help from animism, because the global determinism of the magic

(Marchais 1977) assures them complete healing and complete resolution of their problems. The disturbed people can escape painful situations such as a conflicting relation or an illness, in attributing all their bad things to their possessor. But often, after their healing, the sick people often keep and reinforce their belief in the superstition of possession. It remains an encystement, a magical conviction for the price of the healing. But it is no longer a psychiatric problem, but a socio-cultural one. If society would admit its belief in the fox and his havoc, the sick person could take back his life with no feelings of auto-accusation. The sick person is exempt from responsibility for his bizarre behaviours during his illness. The syndrome of possession is in this sense also a culture-bound syndrome. The fox is a diabolical existence admitted by the Japanese. And possession by the fox is proof that the sick person is not at all responsible for the bad things he does.

References

A) In Japanese:

Daiguji M., Kurokawa Y., Imai T.: Examens cliniques sur les états de possession psychogène et schizophrénique. Rinsho-Seishin-Igaku (Psychiatrie clinique), 1978, 7, (12), 1451-1458.

Ishizuka T.: Les possessions japonaises. Mirai-Sha, Tokyo, 1959.

Kondo Y.: La croyance à Inari. Hanawa-Shobo, Tokyo, 1978.

Kuba M.: A psychopathological and socio-cultural psychiatric study of possession syndrome. Seishin-Shinkeigaku-Zasshi (J. de psychiatrie et neurologie), 1973, 75, (3), 169-186.

Miyamoto T. (a): L'état de possession- au point de vue ethno-psychiatrique. Rinsho - Seishin - Igaku, 1979, 8, (9). Réédition dans: Études des délires et leur frontière. Kobun-do, Tokyo, 1981.

Miyamoto T. (b): Les thèmes délirants schizophréniques - ses spécificités japonaises. Seishin-Igaku, 1979, 21, (2), 143-152. Réédition dans: “Etudes des délires et leur frontière”.

Morita K.: A propos de ce que j’appelle “psychose d’invocation”. Sinkei-Shi (J. de neurologie), 1915, 14, 286-287.

Murakami H.: Sur l’état de possession. Dans: Théories psychopathologiques I, 1971. Cité par Miyamoto (1979 a).

Nishimura K.: Cultural psychiatric studies of possession syndrome in Nambu area. Seishin-Igaku (Psychiatrie), 1976, 18, (12), 1261-1269.

Nisimura K.: L’évolution moderne du chamanisme. Rinsho-Seishin-Igaku, 1977, 6, (12), 1607- 1626.

Nishimura K.: Schizophrénie, Psychose de possession et contexte médical. Dans: Bunretsubyo-No-Seishin Byori VII (Psychopathologies de la schizophrénie). Todai-Todai-Shuppan-Kai, Tokyo, 1978.

Oda S.: Histoire japonaise de la folie. Shisakusha, Tokyo, 1981.

Ogino K.: Considérations psychopathologiques sur l’état de possession. Seishin-Byorigaku-Kenkyu (Recherches psychopathologiques), 1974, 1, 94- 122.

Rhee H.: On reactive psychosis associated with folk-belief in Japan. Seishin-Shinkeigaku-Zasshi, 1961, 63, 296- 310.

Sato T.: Phénomène de possession et psychose d’invocation. Nihon-Iji-Shinpo (Nouvelles médicales japonaises), n. 2667, 125.

Sato S., Sugano K., Takaesu Y., Miyasaka M., Oda S.: On the two cases of frog-possession (batracanthropia). Seishin-Igaku, 1975, 17, (3), 203-252. Avec résume én anglais.

Shinfuku N.: On the Kitsune-Tsuki (possession of demon-foxes) in the San-In district. Seishin-Igaku, 1959, 1, (2), 83-90.

B) In European languages:

Bourgeois M., Broustra J., Favarel-Garrigues B., Hébert A.: A propos des délires de sorcellerie. A.M.P., 1971, 2, (4), 575-592.

Calmeil J.-L.-F.: De la folie considérée sous le point de vue pathologique, philosophique, historique et judiciaire. 2 Vol. Paris, 1845. Réédition par Laffitte, 1982, Marseille.

Delay J.: Délire de possession diabolique - guérison par l'électro-choc. Presse Médicale, 1965, 11, 143.

Marchais P.: Magie et mythe en psychiatrie. Masson, 1977, Paris.

Oesterreich T.K.: Phénoménologie des Ich. Iste bard, 1910. Cité par Daiguji et coll., 1978

Oesterreich T.K.: Les possédés. Payot. Paris, 1929. Cité par Daiguji el coll. 1978 et par Sato et coll. 1975.

Seglas J.: Leçons cliniques sur les maladies mentales et nerveuses. Asselin et Houzean, 1895, Paris.

Yap P.M.: The possession syndrome - a comparison of Hong-Kong and French findings. J. Med. Sci., 1960, 106, 110-137.

Historical Reminiscences: The Schizophrenic Psychosis of the Empress of Mexico

C. Müller

Summary: Quite a number of reports have been published on psychotic developments in the mental make-up of kings and rulers, especially during the past century. Particularly remarkable is the great interest which has been evinced to date on the fate of King Ludwig II of Bavaria. On the other hand, the tragedy of the Belgian Princess Charlotte, who was Empress of Mexico for a few years by the side of her husband, Maximilian of Austria, is hardly known. I could not find anything about her in psychiatric literature, but there are numerous biographical hints in books on history dealing with the dramatic episode of the short-lived Mexican empire. I found some of the most essential information on the personality and psychosis of Empress Charlotte in the book written by Countess H. de Reinach-Foussemange. The following description is necessarily sketchy and should be considered as a preliminary report to a more comprehensive interpretation of Charlotte's personality.

BORN AS THE 3RD CHILD of King Leopard I in 1840, the small princess, until puberty, was described at first as a happy and open, but later as a reflective and deeply religious child. It is not to be overlooked that her father had openly wished for a son, and did not conceal his disappointment at her birth. Her mother gave her up early; already by the age of 16 her marriage had been arranged. By 17 she was married to the archduke Maximilian of Austria.

In the years 1859-1863, Napoleon III's plan gained power. Wanting to form an empire in Mexico, despite warning voices, Maximilian annexed the crown. In 1864 the royal pair landed in Mexico. As countless published letters show, the empress was full of lofty plans, ambitious and progressive, while her husband was publicly restrained. The reading of her letters conveys the impression that Charlotte was filled with the burning desire to give the world proof of her abilities (surely to redeem herself in the eyes of her father). She mixed herself constantly in the inner and outer policies of her country, and was continually occupied with correspondence, while Maximilian primarily concerned himself with ceremonies of the court and protocol questions. Between the lines it can be read that their relationship was not ideal. Maximilian had mistresses, Charlotte, it can be supposed, was frigid.

What had been prophesied, then happened: the French expedition corps, under the leadership of Marshall Bazaine did not succeed in stopping the rebellion under Juarez; Napoleon III must have realized that he was in trouble. The relations between the two ruling houses cooled down; the French expedition corps was called back. In this despairing situation, Charlotte went to find help in Europe, and was in Paris in the summer of 1866. Her conferences with Napoleon III and his partner Eugénie, proved to be useless. Contemporaries reported with what vehemence Charlotte led the conversations; hysterical scenes resulted, in which she threw herself on the floor in St.-Cloud: in a letter to her spouse she threw exalted accusations at Napoleon III: "He wants to commit a bad deed prepared well in advance, not because of cowardice, discouragement, or any other reason, but because he represents the principal of evil in the world and he wants to do away with good, even though humanity does not see the evil of his ways, and adores him."

Bitter, she left Paris and traveled to the Miramare castle in Triest, and from there back to Rome in September of 1866, in order to speak to the Pope. Pius IX received her with much pomp but did not give in to her demand for mediation. In these weeks, the dramatic excitement now appears as the first signs of psychotic manifestation: Charlotte suspected a plot against her, and was convinced someone wanted to poison her. On the occasion of her second visit to Pius IX, a dramatic scene took place, in which she entered his private chambers, and ripped his cup of chocolate out of his hands, expressing that she was dying from hunger, as people everywhere were trying to poison her. She was interrupted passing through the Vatican libraries; then she returned back to her hotel where she left megalomaniacal decrees for the removal of her court position. Only still served by her Austrian servants, she had hens roasted and killed before her eyes, for fear of poisoning; she had a coach drive her through the city of Rome to a public well where she could get drinking water. Doctors were called, her brother, the duke of Flanders, hurried to see her and took her to Miramare castle, and from here on it appears her delusional psychosis took hold of her. She hardly slept any longer, and passed her nights sitting in a chair. She spoke of Maximilian as the bird of the earth and sovereign of the universe. The psychiatrist, Riedel, was called from Vienna. He ordered her complete isolation and so was envisaged Miramare's garden house with locks and secured windows. From here she wrote normal, friendly letters to her acquaintances. The shooting of her husband in June 1867, in Queretaro, was kept from her, and over time she became less and less interested with the events in Mexico. Maximilian was no longer mentioned in her letters. In the same year, 1867, the Belgian court decided to have her brought to them, not without diplomatic difficulties arising in Vienna. Finally, she was brought to Brussels almost with force, where she found her home in the Tervueren tower. The Belgian psychiatrist, Bulkens, who at the time led the famous colony Gheel, cared for her; later it was Dr. Hart.

Many years of a withdrawn life followed. The days passed with knitting, walks, expeditions and conversations. It was apparent in her letters that her behavior changed. While she was quiet and calm, she could suddenly fly into a state of excitation, in which she hit opponents, tore books, and screamed. Letters of the court ladies indicate that there were sometimes difficulties with her nourishment. After much deliberation and delay, the terrible news of her husband's death was broken to her; she reacted with grief and tears, and above all she said she was not capable even of going to confession.

In 1870, in a letter from the Viscount de Conway, it appears that the condition of the empress was not particularly good. "She is without hope. The unhappy princess shall remain deprived of reason." People were astounded by the fact that her bodily health remained good, and she was still very pretty.

Details of her psychotic behavior are naturally not found in her letters to her relatives and ladies of the court. It only appeared in disguised hints. For example: "The life of the unfortunate girl is divided between crises characterized by a destructive monomania and periods of physical calm."

Attention should be drawn to one particular thing in her letters: she never referred to herself in the first person, but instead used "we" or "one"; for example "do not find fault with it, my lord, one is crazy, yes my lord, one is old, one is stupid, one is crazy. The insane woman is still alive." That she publicly, actively hallucinated was evident by the following remarks: during excursions, walks and sitting in the society room, she remained silent most of the time. However, she had lively conversations in German, French and English with "imaginary" conversation partners. What she said appeared to be incoherent, and her monologues were interrupted by laughter here and there. In 1912, on her birthday, she wrote "Maximilian is not here." and "Blücher came in time to save the situation, but in Mexico, nothing, nothing." An unbelievable ambivalence to spouses appeared when she suddenly dramatically stated, "One had a husband, an emperor, a king, a large wedding, my lord. Then madness. My lord, it is the cause of a murder. Maximilian, archduke, Hapsburg house. Villain, fatal. Napoleon a genius, to have reigned."

The ill woman took no more notice of the passing of time or history. The first world war covered Europe with terror, the German army occupied Belgium, she stayed in her tower and outlived most of her contemporaries. The war came to end, and on the 19th of January, 1927, the old empress passed away. A state burial honored her memory.

A following commentary to this story of the ill: a sensitive, somewhat stubborn young person with large fantasies, searches the realization of her dreams through her marriage to a high-ranking, but weak duke, who brought her into a politically failing adventure. She achieved carrying the title of empress at 24, which she held over all her contemporaries. With conventional formulas she tried to gloss over contact difficulties with her duke and threw herself blindly into politics. When the weak building of her glory began to collapse, she turned to the two father figures of her world, Napoleon III and the Pope. Rejected by both, she began to lose contact with reality. The threat of her outer position turned into panic and fear towards her loss of bodily integrity. Oral-sadistic tendencies turned her against herself. A genuine resignation is not possible, for years she supported herself again and again on primitive-aggressive excitement against her destiny. Under the weight of monotony and futility of her existence, her resistance dropped. Without, even speech failed her. She became more and more involved in her isolation, and only in her hallucinations did she play the role of empress.

With these remarks I will break off here, but I would like to give the reader the idea of becoming absorbed in this peculiar story. Who can give information about Dr. Riedel from Vienna? Did he write anything about his contacts with the empress? Who was Dr. Bulkens?

References

Buffin, C.: Les impératrices Charlotte et Eugénie. A. de. Wil Edit: Bruxelles.

Coffin, R.: Charlotte l'impératrice fantome. Edition de France, Paris, 1937.

Praviel, A.: La vie tragique de l'impératrice Charlotte Collection le sphinx, Paris 1930.

de Reinach-Foussemange, H.: Charlotte de Belgique impératrice du Mexique. Librairie Plon, Paris, 1929.

Self-testimony of a schizophrenic around 1800

J. E. Meyer and R. Meyer

Summary: Report on a patient who was treated between 1798 and 1813 at the Bethlem Hospital in London for a paranoic-hallucinatory schizophrenia. There exist detailed self-descriptions by this patient, who was suffering from political persecution mania and megalomania, as well as the reports of his doctors, which were partly published and partly kept on record. He had also made detailed designs of the machine by which he felt himself influenced. This is probably one of the first cases of self-description by a psychotic patient.

THE CASE OF JAMES TILLY MATTHEWS (M.), a mentally ill person, which occurred in the Bethlem Hospital in London between 1798 and 1813, caused a public sensation. With unusual obstinacy his relatives pursued his release for years. The attending doctor and eminent psychiatrist John Haslam (7,8) published a caustic note under the title "Illustrations of Madness"(3), with many quotations from the patient, and the return of his "persecution apparatus". This publication was at the same time a document of justification.

The story of M.'s suffering, readable in his self-description, the judgment of his doctor, and the mentality of his environment, is also remarkable today in various respects; the abrupt descriptions of his psychotic experiences, their explanation and meaning given by the patient himself; the relations of his insane thoughts to the political situation, the position of science and technology at the end of the 18th century and beginning of the 19th century, through which his psychosis characterized an interdependence of persecution and megalomania and finally through the interest of the public. This fundamentally contributed to the fact that his doctors Haslam and Monro fortified their positions after decade - long activities at the Bethlem Hospital (4,8). The descriptions and judgments of Haslam, a psychiatrist of outstanding aptitude, afford a glimpse into the clinical psychiatry of England at the time (8).

This study is based on a handwritten document of the patient (1), on John Haslam's publication (3), and on the statements of Haslam, Thomas Monro, and other doctors at a judicial interrogation on the question of his release from the hospital (2). Further information sources are the protocols of the parliamentary commission of 1815 (4), and the medical reports taken from the records of the hospital. In German literature there is Griesinger's "Illustrations of Madness", and with a reproduction of machine drawings from M. - referred to by F. Nasse in the first edition of the periodical for psychiatric doctors (1818). In this way Krauss should also be mentioned as having knowledge of M.; he mentioned him in "Nothschrie" and was associated with Nasse.

As little is known about M's childhood and youth as about his origins. His birthdate is missing; his age was never known. His mother and a sister appear to have died during his childhood. M. was a resident of London, and tea-broker by career. He was married, visiting rights were taken away from his wife because her pressure for his release was felt to be a bother. M. had two children.

The Politically Paranoid

M. reports (3), that he was detained during his stay in Paris in 1793 until the beginning of 1796 by the French government, and that he was put in different prisons. M. came shortly to the conviction that a plan existed to betray secrets of the British government to France, to proclaim the republic in Britain and Ireland, and to disorganize the British fleet. He became personally occupied with the head of the French security police and his affairs. He was surrounded with police, his letters were held back, and it was sought to hinder his four trips between England and France. He strictly refused to cooperate with French plans to help with magnetic methods. As M. then again in England - went to share his information with the English government, he found himself surrounded by Paris agents (magnetic spy workers), who worked together with London gangs. M. was further convinced that the alleged stolen jewels of the French queen were left to members of the English royal dynasty through bribery, in order to betray England and to separate Scotland and Ireland from England.

According to M., the duke of York, with help from Prussian kings, would become king of France. The Prussian king also planned the destruction of General Washington, in order to establish two English monarchies in America.

It is evident from Haslam's report that M., through these campaigns, believed his fatherland to be in great danger, above all from the French side, as well as his own life being at risk through wanting to avert these dangers. Three months before his admittance to the Bethlem hospital, M. caused a sensation in a hearing at the British House of Commons by calling "treason". He later explained this to Haslam, that he was active as a peace negotiator on the order of the French and English governments, but that he was given no wage and not once were his traveling costs paid for.

The Delusion of Persecution

M. spoke of a gang which was comprised of 4 men and 3 women: schooled in "pneumatic chemistry", who operated a machine he named an "air loom". M. alternated terming the gang workers "assassins, pneumaticians, political chemists, rascals, wretches, villains, monsters" (quote IV). M. gives a description of each member of the gang, not unlike a warrant of arrest, he gives names, ages, height and clothing, language, position in the gang and to the machine. The gang was lead by Bill, the "king". Under his magnetic influence, another patient of the Bethlem hospital, James Hadfield, was to undertake the sensational assassination attempt of King George III, on May 1, 1800. It is suggested that another person, named Sir Archy, was a woman disguised as a man; Sir Archy's speech is full of lies and obscenities. M. believed a girl named Charlotte to be of French descent, and to be held in the gang as a scarcely clothed, malnourished prisoner; some members of the gang did not, (or seldom) work the machine, but established contacts with other gangs, working through "brain saying" or with magnets.

What M. suffered in his psychosis, - this terrible catalogue of human misery - was comprised of a mental impairment and corporal torture, as Haslam named it: under the category of mental impairment - "thought making"; the production of foreign thoughts, "poking"; the paralysis of resistance to mental impairments (through injections of fluid diagonally through the body in the direction of the genitals) (III), "tying down"; the diminution of powers of judgment, "witting soul from sense", in which M. understood a magnetic blockade in the connection between the emotions of the heart and the actions of the intellect. Further to be named are: "brain -" or "voice sayings, hearing voices; "thigh talking", voices noticed coming from his upper thigh and understood by the brain. Also, the production of terrible smells by the machine, in a dream, ("dream working") affected his waking thoughts. Especially detailed was the description of "kiting": as a child lets a kite climb in the air, so also could an assassin, with the help of the machine or through magnetic "impregnation", "lift up" remarkable thoughts in his brain. The afflicted knew constantly that they were not his thoughts, that they originated from the outside, and were "kited". Similarly, there was "brain-lengthening", namely the distortion of particular thoughts. Serious and solemn convictions became laughable through this. M. added that this could actually appear as insanity.

The corporal tortures were as follows: the pulling of the mouth into a grimace ("laugh making"), the appeasement of the genitals with a magnetic fluid; the rolling of the tongue causing a speech impediment; ("eye screwing"); the production of an apoplexy (through the forceful infiltration of fluids into the head); "bomb-bursting" the machine would bring a sort of electric battery steam, gas and fluid to the body in an explosion; "gag-plucking", the sucking at magnetic fluids from the anus; the production of bladder stones or a raw, burning stomach slime; the nailing of the knee joints, and finally the occurrence of sudden death caused by magnetic pressures in the atmosphere which brought circulation to a standstill. M. named this "lobster-cracking".

All sorts of tortures and mental impairments depend on "event working" (IV) and are expressions of "assailment", that is to say attack. The victim is an "assailed person", who works for "event workers" or the "assailing gang" sometimes for years, who has a goal, "the event"."

A closer description of the "air loom" can be foregone in view of it's illustration. M. was of the opinion that the whole machine was portrayed in Chamber's Dictionary of 1783 under the word "loom". A part of the machine, named "music glasses", was illustrated as an electronic battery in an encyclopedia. If it wanted to observe members of the gang, it could interrupt connections to it's victim with a piece of metal, and make itself invisible. M. was convinced that such machines served by a gang were in many places in London. M. gives an example: while the war minister was in church, at home, or in office, the thought "exchange of prisoners" would be produced, and at the same time his French colleagues would obtain information about it. The "air-loom" was applied to people who were first prepared by novices of the gang with "hard-impregnation", and without being able to perceive it, they were made to breathe in a magnetic liquid.

M. characterized "the assassin" as a victim and a talisman. Haslam points out that for M., in spite of all his suffering, something like consolation was present in his relations with the gang workers; through these relations M. was able to discover his thoughts and actions, with his "scientific advances", his resistance also grew. Haslam mentions the triumph M. felt, when through cleverness and unremitting vigilance he escape persecution, while his mother, sister, brother and only son fell victims to the gang, according to his convictions. The assassin let M. know that he and the working machine, "the Bedlam-attaining-airloom-warp" were to be found in a basement opposite the hospital and that a secret exit was found in the old London city wall (the street on which Bethlem hospital was built, was called London Wall). At best, according to him (1), everything should be put under water in order to eliminate it; for shortly Glasgow's psychiatric asylum would be flooded, the patients would cure themselves, and become conspicuously quiet. M. explained that, as in all other "madhouses" in Great Britain, active gang-workers in the basements would be stopped in their criminal activities by the rush of water. The so-called mentally ill were therefore only the poor victims of the "event-worker." (IV)

Megalomania

In the form of a royal decree as "James, Absolute, Sole and Supreme Sacred Omni Imperious Arch Grand Arch Sovereign Arch Proprietor Emperor Supreme", M. made a generous offer to all who wanted to help being usurpers, who were at work in

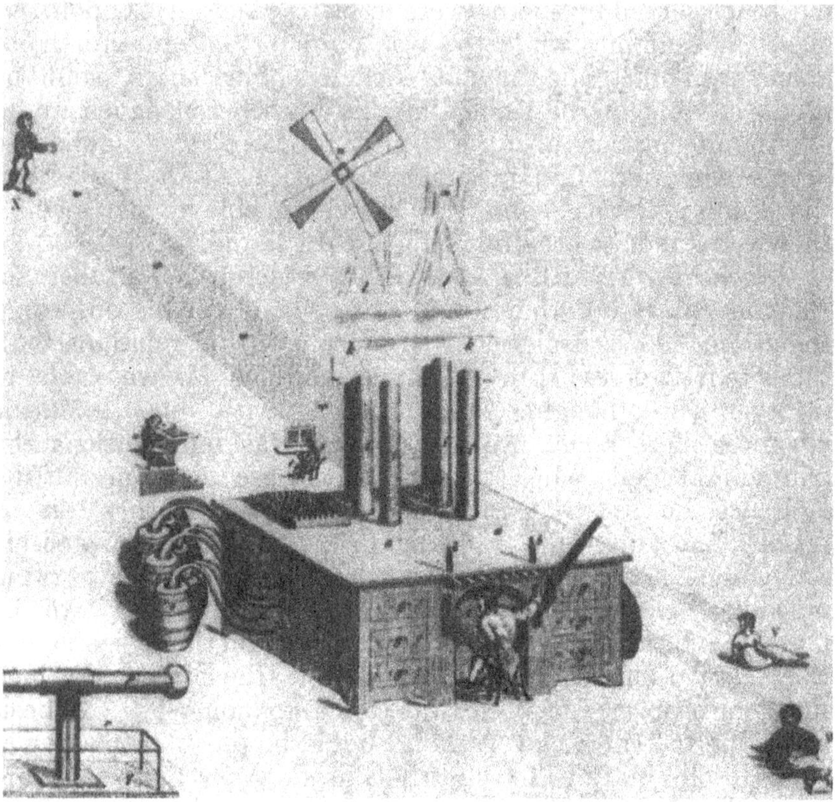

1. Air-loom (pneumatic machine): aa= surface of the apparatus like a large table. bb= metal, in order to interrupt connections to an "assailed person". c= place where the apparatus was to be served. ee= handle for the production of "lobster cracking". h= electric battery on the table for "bomb bursting". iklm= upper part of the machine, not clearly recognized by M. o= container for magnetic gas. pqr= made of brass, no explanation. ss= wires to conduct magnetic fluids to an "assailed person". x= could be made to turn different colors when heated. t= switch for repetition and strengthening of inspection. u= Jack the school master, one of the gang workers who changed M's speaking and writing. v= Charlotte. W= Sir Archy.

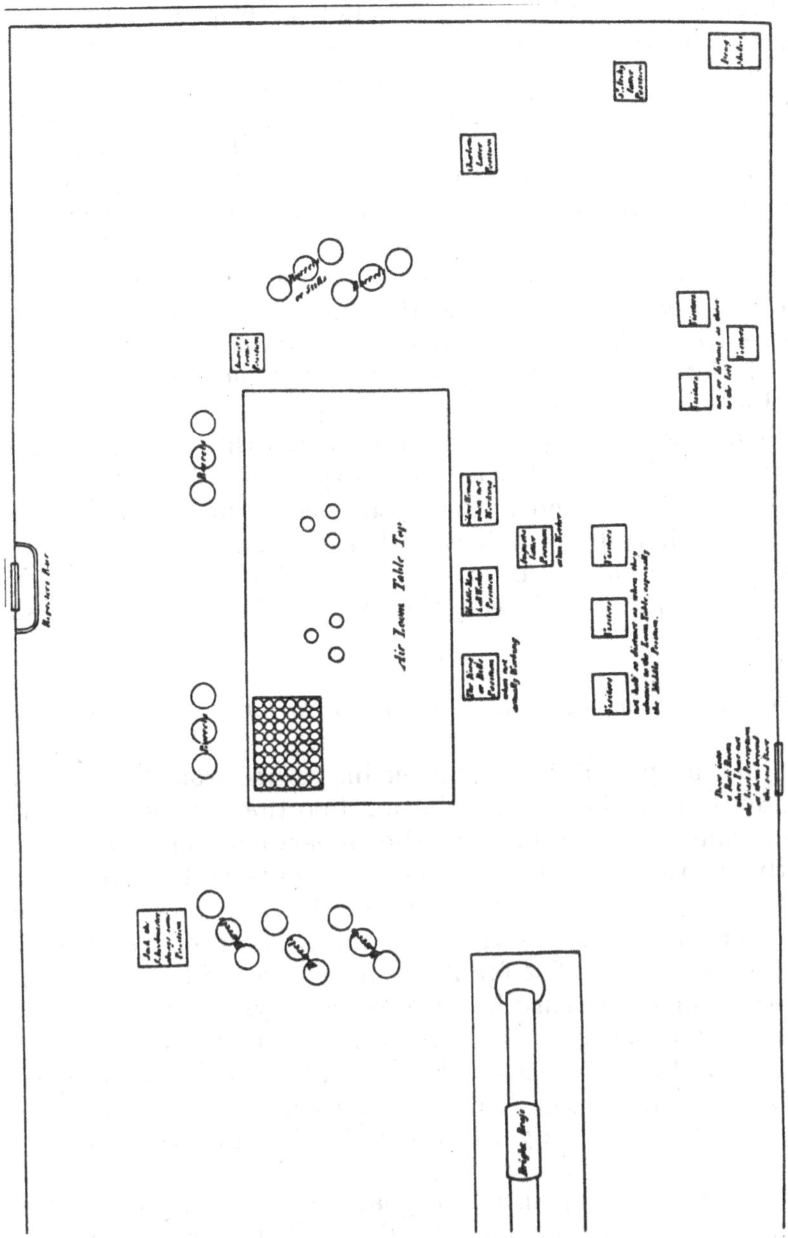

2. Ground drawing of the air-loom

many countries, into his power, by offering rewards of a million pounds. He wanted usurpers to be brought to him living, so that he could hand or behead them (IV). Their machines should be handled over undestroyed, in order to be made known to the public. If servants of the usurpers abandoned them immediately, they should not be punished. M. counted all usurpers deserving death to be not only the gang workers, but also all government officials in France and England, and in England also all parliamentarians, bankers, and above all the royal family with king George III at its head, whom he named "George Guelph". His vengeance went farther, to the entire staff of Bethlem, ministers, police and judges in connection with his forced hospitalization. M. spoke of his subjects as "good subjects" and expected them to testify that their absolute sovereign had been born. He explained that all land, possessions, power and authority in the world had originally belonged to his family and was therefore rightfully his since birth. There is also talk of "Her Omni Arch Majesty" in his documents, whose life was threatened three times by an assassin.

Matthew's Case in the Judgment of his Doctors

On January 1, 1798, soon after his return from France, M. was admitted to the Bethlem hospital on the suggestion of his parish, and one year later to the department of incurables. Shortly before his death in 1810 he was on leave from Bethlem and in the private care home of Mr. Fox in Hackney "for a change of air"; he never witnessed the removal of his doctors, Haslam and Monro. The family, from the time of his admission on, strove for his release in all possible ways. This led to the patient being brought to a hearing in 1799 before Lloyd Kenyon, Lord Chief Justice of England (2). The family pursued a new proposal for his dismissal in 1809. At this time, two hospital doctors secretly examined M. who appeared perfectly healthy.

The hospital appointed a board of doctors under the guidance of the president of the Royal College of Physicians, Sir Lucas Pepys, with another examination of the patient. The eight doctors were in complete agreement that M. was mentally ill and dangerous for his environment, especially for the royal family. There is a letter to Whitehall, dated the 7th of August, 1809, from Lord Liverpool, the Interior minister of the time, which recommends the further detainment of the patient, and the costs of his stay and his grave in case of his death were to be taken over. (2)

> In the course of time, M. enjoyed many advantages over other sick, he had his own furniture in his room, including a chair which he considered to be his throne (4). For his plans for the erection of a new Bethlem hospital, he received 30 Guineas from the governor of the hospital. John Haslam was especially interested in him, and let him learn copper engraving through one of his friends.

In the unabridged quote (VII), in many regards remarkable summaries of the governor of Bethlem hospital (2) say that regardless of exceptional difficulties which this patient went through over the course of many years in the hospital, his release could not be recommended on consideration of the king, the public, the sick, and his friends. In fact, above all, death threats against the king up until shortly before his death, hindered his release.

On the occasion of the juridical decision about M's release, Haslam was listened to in detail; he knew M's tribunal in advance, and that a description of his megalomania would be referred to. According to Haslam (2,3), M. was convinced that Bethlem's drinking water was poisoned, he suffered from pain in his joints, because someone had mixed substances with chemical or magnetic effects in with his food. M. refused to speak with other patients, because they were only tools against his judicial intrigues. M. thought he saw a figure on the tower of the neighboring church of Bloomsbury, who carried the Doomsday Book under his arm.

Discussion

We are dealing here with a paranoid-hallucinatory schizophrenia. The diagnosis gives no difficulties; next to perceptions of delusion (for example the Doomsday Book figure) and influencing experiences, there are suggested thoughts, "brain and voice-sayings", hallucinations of smell, and optical illusions.

Clear-cut new word formations are lacking. The symptomology of the sick person has apart from the content of the delusions - after more than 150 years, nothing to differentiate it from a schizophrenic of today.

> The characteristic changing of delusion and hallucination is evident in the following example: M. understood that as he came through Holborn, the Lord Chancellor, saw, how several people wanted to kill an alleged rabies-ridden dog. The voices of the persecutor report: "It is as you say: we pursue you, we meet you with our murder intentions." The Lord Chancellor found no trace of rabies in the dog, held it up in his arms, and freed it from the enraged people. He gave instructions to put it in the stables and have it cared for. Again came the voices of the persecutor: "Yes, this is a mockery: he cares for the dog, but you are damned, and must lie in the stables." M. added that "lying in the stable" was a customary expression for admitting someone into Bethlem's "incurable" department.

The psychosis took a chronic course. The treating doctors, Monro and Haslam, in 1809, stressed that, M., over the course of ten years, never once distanced himself from his delusions. Delusions of pursuit and megalomania underwent an increasing expansion, and a systemization, as Haslam remarked. Both domains further developed during his long hospitalization, with reciprocal influences. Haslam began his "Illustrations of Madness" with the ascertainment that M. behaved sometimes like a robot in the hands of agents, and sometimes like the ruler of the world, dispensing proclamations to his untrue subjects.

The content of the delusions of the pursued are the political themes of the time; namely a state of war between France and England, with a short 22 year interval; on the explanation of pursuit in technical delusion - magnetism and electricity were called upon, where these methods of influence were effectively looked at constantly over the organic substratum; the brain. M.'s omnipotent images at the time had a clearly archaic form. One can also calculate what M. understood from the voices of his pursuers in reference to his relations with Napoleon: he was Bonaparte's talisman. The event worker would lift Bonaparte to highest glory through M., but degrade M. to a subhuman degree.

There is no writing which M. publicized himself. In the "Illustrations of Madness", Haslam mentioned a manuscript of M.'s which he quoted; M. was thankful for the communication of his conceptions in an open-minded publication.

In the comparison of J.T. Matthews case with "Cry of distress of a magnetically poisoned" (5), it is recognized that the technical delusion of M. and Krauss, even though it is separated by a half century, shows many similarities, above all in regard to magnetic influences. While Krauss, to be sure, only had a negligible interest in the machine's pursual, it's representation, description, and illustration played a large roll to M. From the air-loom's magnets, fine lines led to an "impregnated" person, which were full of a liquid causing sympathy, attraction to repulsion, comparable to the effects of magnets according to their positions to the poles. With a distance of over 1000 feet, the "fluid-wires" would rip and their influence would therefore cease.

Krauss's psychosis - a hypochondriatic paraphrenia according to Leonhard - also developed chronic disorder without remission. With Krauss, as with M., the first signs of illness became visible during a trip: without the details of a connection between the outbreak of psychosis and a foreign sojourn being known. If Krauss, after his 1 1/2 year stay in the Celitten monastery in Antwerp, did not require further stationary treatment, it primarily fits that he would have felt to be delivered from his pursuers, and no vengeance plans (pursuing the pursuers) or megalomania would have developed. His defense consisted of - apart from his virtuous abilities - fleeing his pursuers - in efforts to enlighten the public and on the request of the doctors - in order to free himself from the effects of magnetism. Both M. and Krauss, in contrast to Schreber and Staudenmeyer, saw what would happen to them only in negative terms; that holds valid in spite of M.'s megalomania. Neither of them ever showed any sort of understanding of, or insight into, their illness. It remains remarkable, that nevertheless both, in spite of all signs of insanity, in no way clearly rejected their healthy contemporaries. Krauss, during his 50-year hallucinatory psychosis led the life of a relatively successful traveling salesman. M., however - after fifteen years in the "incurable department" of the Bethlem hospital - understood the interest of the public, the government, and the parliament to control him.

Quotes

I. Egyptian snuff: "This disgusting odour is exclusively employed during sleep, when, by their dream-workings, they have placed him, as a solitary wanderer, in the marshes near the mouth of the river Nile...The eye is likewise equally disgusted with the face of the country, which is made to assume a hateful tinge, resembling the dirty and cold blue of a scorbutic ulcer. From this cheerless scene they suddenly awake him, when he finds his nostrils stuffed, his mouth furred, and himself nearly choked by the poisonous effects of their Egyptian snuff"(Haslam, 3)

II. Lobster-cracking: "I do not know any better way for a person to comprehend the general nature of such lobster-cracking operation, than by supposing himself in a sufficiently large pair of nut-crackers or lobster-crackers, with teeth, which should pierce as well as press him through every particle within and without; he experiencing the whole stress, torture, driving, oppressing, and crush all together" (Matthews, 3)

III. Poking: "This magic touch disarms the expression of his resentment, and leaves him an impotent prey to the malignity of their scorn and ridicules" (Haslam, 3)

IV. Event-working: "To show what the nature of such event-working is, namely, how infamous human beings, making a profession of pneumatic chemistry, and pneumatic magnetism, hire themselves as spies; and by impregnating persons, singled out by them as objects for interfering with, obtaining their secrets, actuating them in various ways, in thought, word and deed, as well as they can, to model their conduct, ideas or measures..." (Matthews, 3)

V. "These assassins are so superlatively skilfull in every thing which related to pneumatic chemistry, physiology, nervous influence, sympathy, human mind, and the higher metaphysic, that whenever their persons shall be discovered, and their machine exhibited, the wisest professors will be astonished at their progress, and feel ashamed at their own ignorance." (Haslam, 3)

VI. "It is with Me a Great Object to have them delivered up to Me alive and in their Perfect Senses, And to have their Apparatus unbroken Very whole and in the state they used it, with their Modes etc. Publickly Exhibited" (Matthews, 1)

VII. "If the Judge shall now be satisfied that he ought to discharge the Patient the Governors will be perfectly satisfied also. Far from us having any Interest in his detention their very constitution as one of charity renders it their obvious interest to keep the number of such unhappy Persons as low as possible; and the very great and most improper trouble occasioned for many years past both to the Governors and Officers by the detention of this particular Patient renders his discharge truly desirable. The Governors however are not unmindful that they have a serious duty to perform by the Sovereign and the public as well as by the Patients and their friends and they have therefore pursued the line of conduct which the above Affidavits will explain and (it is hoped) will justify." (2)

References

1. Handgeschriebene Aufzeichnungen (1804). Archives of Bethlem Royal Hospital London.

2. Brief on Rule in the matter of James Tilly Matthews, a Lunatic (1809). Archives of Bethlem Royal Hospital London.

3. Haslam, John: Illustrations of Madness. G. Hayden, London 1810: British Museum.

4. Parliamentary committee appointed to consider of provisions being made for the better regulation of madhouses in England (1815). Archives of Bethlem Royal Hospital London.

5. Ahlenstiehl, H. und Meyer, J. E.: Nothschrei eines magnetisch Vergifteten (Bayer, Leverkusen 1967).

6. Griesinger, W.: Pathologie und Therapie der psychischen Krankheiten (Stuttgart 1861).

7. Leigh, D.: John Haslam, M.D.- 1764-1844. J. Hist. Med. 10: 17-43 (1955).

8. Leigh, D.: The historical development of British psychiatry. I. (Pergamon Press, Oxford 1961).

9. Leonhard, K.: Schizophrene mit typischen Defektzuständen nach ihren eigenen Schriftstücken. Arch. Psychiat. 211: 7-22 (1968).

10. Nasse, F.: In Zeitschr. f. psychische Ärzte, Bd. 1 (Cnobloch, Leipzig 1818).

11. O'Donoghue, E. G.: The story of Bethlem Hospital (Dutton, New York 1915).

12. Schreber, D.P.: Denkwürdigkeiten eines Nervenkranken (Mutze, Leipzig 1903).

13. Staudenmaier, L.: Die Magie als experimentelle Naturwissenschaft (Akad. Verlagses., Leipzig 1912).

THE RESHAPING OF PSYCHOANALYSIS
From Sigmund Freud to Ernest Becker

This series is designed to offer works which are concerned with the reshaping and revitalization of psychoanalysis. Also critical to this series is the interweaving of such disciplines as psychology, psychiatry, religion, and philosophy so as to promote dialogue and offer avenues toward rapprochement.

This series will publish and proffer studies of Freud and Neo-Freudians such as Becker which are most aware of the long term contributions of psychoanalysis toward the healing of self and society. Studies should be scholarly and clinically discerning. This is a series which is keenly concerned with the bridging of disciplines, the networking of ideas and peoples, and with the perpetuation of the psychoanalytic questions, and, at times, its answers. This is a series which is also very open to its authors' creativity and most appreciative of those efforts which reshape, revamp, revitalize, and transform Freudian psychoanalysis.

The general series editor is Barry R. Arnold, an Emory Ph.D., who is Associate Professor of Religious Studies and Philosophy at the University of West Florida. His speciality area is psychoanalysis and medical ethics.

Barry R. Arnold
5820 Kirkland Drive
Milton, FL 32570
(904) 474-2066